# Non-Invasive Technologies for the Diagnosis and Management of Skin Cancer

*Editors*

AARON S. FARBERG
DARRELL S. RIGEL

# DERMATOLOGIC CLINICS

www.derm.theclinics.com

*Consulting Editor*
BRUCE H. THIERS

October 2017 • Volume 35 • Number 4

**ELSEVIER**

1600 John F. Kennedy Boulevard • Suite 1800 • Philadelphia, Pennsylvania, 19103-2899

http://www.theclinics.com

**DERMATOLOGIC CLINICS Volume 35, Number 4**
**October 2017 ISSN 0733-8635, ISBN-13: 978-0-323-54662-1**

Editor: Jessica McCool
Developmental Editor: Sara Watkins

*Dermatologic Clinics* (ISSN 0733-8635) is published quarterly by Elsevier Inc., 360 Park Avenue South, New York, NY 10010-1710. Months of publication are January, April, July, and October. Business and editorial offices: 1600 John F. Kennedy Blvd., Suite 1800, Philadelphia, PA 19103-2899. Customer service office: 11830 Westline Drive, St. Louis, MO 63146. Periodicals postage paid at New York, NY, and additional mailing offices. Subscription prices are USD 377.00 per year for US individuals, USD 655.00 per year for US institutions, USD 434.00 per year for Canadian individuals, USD 799.00 per year for Canadian institutions, USD 505.00 per year for international individuals, USD 799.00 per year for international institutions, USD 100.00 per year for US students/residents, and USD 240.00 per year for Canadian and international students/residents. International air speed delivery is included in all *Clinics* subscription prices. All prices are subject to change without notice. **POSTMASTER:** Send address changes to *Dermatologic Clinics*, Elsevier Health Sciences Division, Subscription Customer Service, 3251 Riverport Lane, Maryland Heights, MO 63043. **Customer Service: 1-800-654-2452 (U.S. and Canada); 314-447-8871 (outside U.S. and Canada). Fax: 314-447-8029. E-mail: journalscustomerservice-usa@elsevier.com (for print support); journalsonlinesupport-usa@elsevier.com (for online support).**

*Reprints.* For copies of 100 or more, of articles in this publication, please contact the Commercial Reprints Department, Elsevier Inc., 360 Park Avenue South, New York, New York 10010-1710. Tel.: 212-633-3874; Fax: 212-633-3820; Email: reprints@elsevier.com.

The *Dermatologic Clinics* is covered in *MEDLINE/PubMed (Index Medicus)*, *Current Contents/Clinical Medicine*, *Excerpta Medica*, *Chemical Abstracts*, and *ISI/BIOMED*.

# Contributors

## CONSULTING EDITOR

**BRUCE H. THIERS, MD**
Professor and Chairman, Department of
Dermatology and Dermatologic Surgery,
Medical University of South Carolina,
Charleston, South Carolina, USA

## EDITORS

**AARON S. FARBERG, MD**
Resident, Department of Dermatology, Icahn
School of Medicine at Mount Sinai, New York,
New York, USA

**DARRELL S. RIGEL, MD, MS**
Clinical Professor, Department of
Dermatology, NYU School of Medicine,
New York, New York, USA

## AUTHORS

**ROBERT L. BARD, MD, DABR, FASLM**
Director, Bard Cancer Center; Founder,
Biofoundation for Angiogenesis Research;
Diplomate, American Board of Radiology;
Fellow, American Society of Lasers in Medicine
and Surgery; Member, International Society of
Dermatologic Surgery, New York, New York,
USA

**BRIAN BERMAN, MD, PhD**
Professor, Department of Dermatology,
University of Miami Miller School of Medicine,
Aventura, Florida, USA

**JULIANA BERK-KRAUSS, BA**
Medical Student, Yale School of Medicine,
New Haven, Connecticut, USA; Research
Fellow, The Ronald O. Perelman Department of
Dermatology, NYU School of Medicine,
New York, New York, USA

**RALPH P. BRAUN, MD**
Department of Dermatology, University
Hospital Zürich, Zürich, Switzerland

**ELIZABETH CHAO, MD, PhD**
Dermatology Resident, Department of
Dermatology, University of Pittsburgh Medical
Center, Pittsburgh, Pennsylvania, USA

**CLAY J. COCKERELL, MD**
Clinical Professor, Department of
Dermatology, The University of Texas
Southwestern Medical Center, Dallas, Texas,
USA

**ELIZABETH D. DRUGGE, PhD, MPH**
Department of Epidemiology and Community
Health, New York Medical College School
of Health Sciences and Practice, Valhalla,
New York, USA

**RHETT J. DRUGGE, MD**
Sheard & Drugge, PC, Stamford Hospital,
Stamford, Connecticut, USA

**REINHARD DUMMER, MD**
Department of Dermatology, University
Hospital Zürich, Zürich, Switzerland

**AARON S. FARBERG, MD**
Resident, Department of Dermatology, Icahn
School of Medicine at Mount Sinai, New York,
New York, USA

**LAURA K. FERRIS, MD, PhD**
Associate Professor, Department of
Dermatology, School of Medicine, University of
Pittsburgh, Pittsburgh, Pennsylvania, USA

**LARS FRENCH, MD**
Department of Dermatology, University
Hospital Zürich, Zürich, Switzerland

**ALEX M. GLAZER, MD**
Resident, Division of Dermatology, Department
of Medicine, University of Arizona College of
Medicine – Tucson, Tucson, Arizona, USA;
National Society for Cutaneous Medicine,
New York, New York, USA

**GARY GOLDENBERG, MD**
Assistant Clinical Professor, Department of
Dermatology, Mount Sinai Medical Center,
New York, New York, USA

**SIMONE GOLDINGER, MD**
Department of Dermatology, University
Hospital Zürich, Zürich, Switzerland

**ATTIYA HAROON, MD, PhD**
Department of Dermatology, Rutgers-Robert
Wood Johnson Medical School, Somerset,
New Jersey, USA

**WHITNEY A. HIGH, MD, JD**
Associate Professor, Department of
Dermatology and Pathology, Director of
Dermatopathology, University of Colorado
School of Medicine, Aurora, Colorado, USA

**SUNIL KALIA, MD MHSc**
Photomedicine Institute, Department of
Dermatology and Skin Science, Vancouver
Coastal Health Research Institute, The
University of British Columbia, Imaging Unit,
Integrative Oncology Department, The BC
Cancer Agency Research Center, Vancouver,
British Columbia, Canada

**VESELINA B. KORCHEVA, MD**
Assistant Professor, Department of
Dermatology, Oregon Health & Science
University, Portland, Oregon, USA

**ROSSITZA LAZOVA, MD**
Director of Dermatopathology, California Skin
Institute, San Jose, California, USA

**SANCY A. LEACHMAN, MD, PhD**
Director, Melanoma and Skin Cancer Program,
Professor and Chair, Department of
Dermatology, OHSU Knight Cancer Institute,
Oregon Health & Science University, Portland,
Oregon, USA

**NAYOUNG LEE, MD**
Department of Dermatology and Cutaneous
Surgery, University of Miami Miller School of
Medicine, Miami, Florida, USA

**AMANDA LEVINE, MD**
Department of Dermatology, SUNY Downstate
Medical Center, Department of Dermatology,
VA NY Harbor Health Care System, Brooklyn,
New York, USA; Department of Dermatology,
Mount Sinai Medical Center, New York,
New York, USA

**KONSTANTINOS LIOPYRIS, MD**
Memorial Sloan Kettering Cancer Center,
New York, New York, USA

**HARVEY LUI, MD**
Photomedicine Institute, Professor and Head,
Department of Dermatology and Skin Science,
Vancouver Coastal Health Research Institute,
The University of British Columbia, Imaging
Unit, Integrative Oncology Department, The BC
Cancer Agency Research Center, Vancouver,
British Columbia, Canada

**JOHANNA MANGANA, MD**
Department of Dermatology, University
Hospital Zürich, Zürich, Switzerland

**MICHAEL A. MARCHETTI, MD**
Memorial Sloan Kettering Cancer Center,
New York, New York, USA

**ASHFAQ A. MARGHOOB, MD**
Attending Physician, Dermatology Service,
Department of Medicine, Memorial Sloan
Kettering Cancer Center, New York,
New York, USA

**ORIT MARKOWITZ, MD**
Assistant Professor, Department of
Dermatology, SUNY Downstate Medical
Center, Department of Dermatology, VA NY
Harbor Health Care System, Brooklyn, New
York, USA; Department of Dermatology, Mount
Sinai Medical Center, New York, New York,
USA

**CHELSEA K. MEENAN, BS**
Medical Student, School of Medicine,
University of Pittsburgh, Pittsburgh,
Pennsylvania, USA

**STEPHANIE MENGDEN KOON, MD**
Assistant Professor, Department of
Dermatology, Oregon Health & Science
University, Portland, Oregon, USA

**DAVID M. PARISER, MD**
Professor, Department of Dermatology,
Eastern Virginia Medical School, Norfolk,
Virginia, USA

**DAVID POLSKY, MD, PhD**
Alfred W. Kopf, MD Professor of
Dermatologic Oncology, The Ronald O.
Perelman Department of Dermatology,
NYU School of Medicine, New York,
New York, USA

**HAROLD RABINOVITZ, MD**
Voluntary Clinical Professor of Dermatology,
Department of Dermatology and Cutaneous
Surgery, University of Miami Miller School of
Medicine, Miami, Florida, USA; Private
Practice, Skin and Cancer Associates,
Plantation, Florida, USA

**BABAR K. RAO, MD, FAAD**
Department of Dermatology, Rutgers-Robert
Wood Johnson Medical School, Somerset,
New Jersey, USA

**DARRELL S. RIGEL, MD, MS**
Clinical Professor, Department of
Dermatology, NYU School of Medicine,
New York, New York, USA

**TOVA ROGERS, MFA**
Memorial Sloan Kettering Cancer Center,
New York, New York, USA

**THEODORE ROSEN, MD**
Professor, Department of Dermatology, Baylor
College of Medicine, Houston, Texas, USA

**ALON SCOPE, MD**
Department of Dermatology, Sheba Medical
Center, Sackler School of Medicine, Tel Aviv
University, Tel Aviv, Israel

**ERIN H. SEELEY, PhD**
Clinical Imaging Principal Investigator, Protea
Biosciences, Inc, Morgantown, West Virginia,
USA

**SHAHRAM SHAFI, MD**
Department of Dermatology, Rutgers-Robert
Wood Johnson Medical School, Somerset,
New Jersey, USA

**DANIEL M. SIEGEL, MD, MS**
Clinical Professor, Department of
Dermatology, SUNY Downstate Medical
Center, Brooklyn, New York, USA

**ARTHUR J. SOBER, MD**
Professor, Department of Dermatology,
Harvard Medical School, Boston,
Massachusetts, USA

**JENNIFER A. STEIN, MD, PhD**
Associate Professor, The Ronald O. Perelman
Department of Dermatology, NYU School of
Medicine, New York, New York, USA

**TRILOKRAJ TEJASVI, MBBS, MD**
Assistant Professor, Director Teledermatology
Services, Department of Dermatology,
University of Michigan, Ann Arbor, Michigan,
USA

**FRANCES M. WALOCKO, MSE, MD**
University of Michigan Medical School,
Ann Arbor, Michigan, USA

**KATIE WANG, DO**
Department of Dermatology, SUNY Downstate
Medical Center, Department of Dermatology,
VA NY Harbor Health Care System, Brooklyn,
New York, USA; Department of Dermatology,
Mount Sinai Medical Center, New York,
New York, USA

**KEVIN P. WHITE, MD**
Associate Professor, Department of
Dermatology, Oregon Health & Science
University, Portland, Oregon, USA

**RICHARD R. WINKELMANN, DO**
Resident, Department of Dermatology,
OhioHealth, Athens, Ohio, USA; Department
of Dermatology, OhioHealth, Columbus,
Ohio, USA

**ZACHARY J. WOLNER, BA**
Memorial Sloan Kettering Cancer Center,
New York, New York, USA

**ORIOL YÉLAMOS, MD**
Memorial Sloan Kettering Cancer Center,
New York, New York, USA

**HAISHAN ZENG, PhD**
Photomedicine Institute, Department of
Dermatology and Skin Science, Vancouver
Coastal Health Research Institute, The
University of British Columbia, Imaging Unit,
Integrative Oncology Department, The BC
Cancer Agency Research Center, Vancouver,
British Columbia, Canada

**JIANHUA ZHAO, PhD**
Photomedicine Institute, Department of
Dermatology and Skin Science, Vancouver
Coastal Health Research Institute, The
University of British Columbia, Imaging Unit,
Integrative Oncology Department, The BC
Cancer Agency Research Center, Vancouver,
British Columbia, Canada

# Contents

and remote US counties where melanoma mortality is doubled for lack of access to dermatologists. Furthermore, serial melanoma screening strategies, serial total body photography, and serial digital dermatoscopy imaging may be performed as a tele-health service, and thus, would be available in any location that can support activity compliant with the Health Insurance Portability and Accountability Act and has appropriate bandwidth.

## Noninvasive Technologies for the Diagnosis of Cutaneous Melanoma

Richard R. Winkelmann, Aaron S. Farberg, Alex M. Glazer, and Darrell S. Rigel

Multispectral analysis devices assess pigmented lesion disorganization at different levels using variable wavelengths of light. Computerized algorithms measure morphologic disorganization of the pigmented skin lesion. Aggregated data of 855 participants investigating the influence of multispectral digital skin lesion analysis (MSDSLA) on practitioner decisions to biopsy pigmented skin lesions revealed the overall sensitivity for detection of melanoma improved from 70% to 88%. Participant specificity increased from 52% to 58% after MSDSLA. Five studies using spectro-photometric intracutaneous analysis scope to evaluate suspicious pigmented skin lesions demonstrated an overall sensitivity and specificity of 85% and 81%, respec-tively, for the detection of melanoma.

## Using Reflectance Confocal Microscopy in Skin Cancer Diagnosis

Attiya Haroon, Shahram Shafi, and Babar K. Rao

Biopsy and histologic evaluation have been the gold standard to diagnose skin tu-mors. Reflectance confocal microcopy (RCM) is a noninvasive, innovative diagnostic technique that enables visualization of different skin layers at an almost histologic resolution. RCM has been proven beneficial in management of various cutaneous lesions. This article highlights the clinical significance and future of RCM to diagnose common skin cancers. However, RCM cannot replace currently standard histopath-ologic diagnosis. More studies are required to better compare the sensitivity and specificity of skin cancer diagnosis using RCM.

## Optical Coherence Tomography in the Diagnosis of Skin Cancer

Amanda Levine, Katie Wang, and Orit Markowitz

Optical coherence tomography (OCT) has emerged as a novel noninvasive imaging device that allows for the real-time, in vivo, cross-sectional imaging of skin morphology. OCT has increased imaging depth and field of view compared with reflectance confocal microscopy, at the cost of decreased cellular resolution. Fre-quency domain OCT, dynamic OCT (D-OCT), and high-definition OCT (HD-OCT) are useful in the diagnosis, treatment planning, and treatment monitoring of nonme-lanoma skin cancers. Research is currently underway to assess the utilization of these devices in distinguishing between malignant and benign melanocytic lesions based on vascular patterns on D-OCT and cellular information on HD-OCT.

## Electrical Impedance Spectroscopy in Skin Cancer Diagnosis

Ralph P. Braun, Johanna Mangana, Simone Goldinger, Lars French, Reinhard Dummer, and Ashfaq A. Marghoob

Electrical impedance spectroscopy (EIS) is a noninvasive method that aims to help diagnose skin cancer. The EIS device consists of a handheld probe with a dispos-able electrode that is applied directly on the skin and uses electrical impendence differences to differentiate between normal and abnormal skin lesions. The EIS algorithm is best used on lesions that are deemed clinically or dermoscopically suspicious and has a high sensitivity in detecting malignant melanoma. The greatest usefulness of EIS is achieved in conjunction with a physician who has experience with this modality and excellent training in the clinical detection of suspicious lesions.

Epidermal genetic information retrieval is a noninvasive diagnostic method involving the application of adhesive tape onto the skin's surface to recover genomic material from the epidermis. This genomic material can then be used in assays to determine gene expression profiles. Studies have shown the potential of this technology to aid clinicians in differentiating between melanomas and nevi. Although this technology is not meant to replace a biopsy, it can help guide the decision whether to biopsy.

The assessment of melanoma by light microscopy with hematoxylin-eosin staining remains an often subjective process. However, there are additional diagnostic measures that may be of utility, such as immunohistochemical staining and genetic evaluation. Adjunctive genetic assessment to augment the diagnosis of melanoma includes comparative genomic hybridization or fluorescent in situ hybridization to assess for gains or losses in genetic material, or gene expression profiling in some form, to ascertain the expression of genes associated with malignancy. Although these techniques may bolster the dermatopathologic assessment of melanoma, none of them, at the present time, are singularly diagnostic. Additional developments in the genetic assessment and prognostication of melanoma are anticipated.

Most melanocytic tumors can be characterized as a benign nevus or a melanoma by a trained pathologist using traditional histopathological methods. However, a minority demonstrates ambiguous features and continues to be a diagnostic challenge. Genetic expression profiling (GEP) assays have been developed in an effort to resolve this dilemma. These assays measure mRNA levels of specified genes using reverse transcription–quantitative polymerase chain reaction technology. The development of GEP assays, methodology, challenges associated with GEP validation and testing, and the suitability of a currently available GEP test for clinical use are reviewed.

A 31-genetic expression profile (31-GEP) test (DecisionDx-Melanoma, Castle Biosciences Inc, Friendswood, TX, USA) was developed as a diagnostic test to assist physicians in the management of cutaneous malignant melanoma. Based on a patient's primary tumor expression levels of a panel of genes (28 discriminating genes and 3 control genes), a lesion is classified as "low risk" (class 1) or "high risk" (class 2) for metastasis. Studies evaluating the clinical utility and impact of the 31-GEP test showed it positively influenced clinical management and patient care, as clinicians incorporated the additional data to modify their clinical recommendations in a risk-appropriate manner.

With the advancement of mobile technologies, smartphone applications (apps) have become widely available and gained increasing attention as a novel tool to deliver dermatologic care. This article presents a review of various apps for skin monitoring and melanoma detection and a discussion of current limitations in the field of dermatology. Concerns regarding quality, transparency, and reliability have emerged because there are currently no established quality standards or regulatory oversight of mobile medical apps. Only a few apps have been evaluated clinically. Further research is needed to evaluate the utility and efficacy of smartphone apps in skin cancer screening and early melanoma detection.

Frances M. Walocko and Trilokraj Tejasvi

Teledermatology has drawn interest in the dermatologic community, because it allows for earlier detection of skin cancer in patients with poor access to health care. Using a combination of dermoscopy and digital photography, teledermatology has demonstrated acceptable concordance with face-to-face clinical diagnoses in multiple settings for pigmented skin lesions. Additional studies on using teledermatology to assess nonpigmented skin lesions are needed. Future advances in mobile teledermatology may help make this technology more widespread and affordable. Although teledermatology is not a replacement for regular total body skin examinations, it is a useful tool to significantly reduce the burden of dermatologic malignancies.

Richard R. Winkelmann, Aaron S. Farberg, Alex M. Glazer, Clay J. Cockerell, Arthur J. Sober, Daniel M. Siegel, Sancy A. Leachman, Whitney A. High, Orit Markowitz, Brian Berman, David M. Pariser, Gary Goldenberg, Theodore Rosen, and Darrell S. Rigel

Early diagnosis and treatment of melanoma improve survival. New technologies are emerging that may augment the diagnosis, assessment, and management of melanoma, but penetrance into everyday practice is low. In the current health care climate, greater emphasis will be placed on the incorporation of technology for clinically suspicious pigmented lesions to facilitate better, more cost-effective management.

# DERMATOLOGIC CLINICS

**THE CLINICS ARE AVAILABLE ONLINE!**
Access your subscription at:
www.theclinics.com

# Erratum

An error was made in the July 2017 issue of *Dermatologic Clinics* (Volume 35, Issue 3) on page 341 of the article, "Long-Term Treatment of Atopic Dermatitis," by James C. Prezzano and Lisa A. Beck. The title of Box 6, "What is the literature for topical corticosteroids use?" should read "What is the literature lacking for topical corticosteroids use?" The online version of the article has been corrected.

Dermatol Clin 35 (2017) xiii
http://dx.doi.org/10.1016/j.det.2017.08.001

# Preface
# The Importance of Early Recognition of Skin Cancer

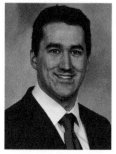  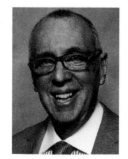

Aaron S. Farberg, MD   Darrell S. Rigel, MD, MS
*Editors*

Skin cancer is the most commonly diagnosed malignancy, with its annual incidence greater than that of all other forms of human malignancy combined. Nearly 5 million people are treated annually in the United States for skin cancer, with an estimated cost of over 8 billion dollars per year. Over 150,000 of those people are diagnosed with melanoma, the deadliest form of skin cancer, each year. Although a massive public health initiative is underway to help educate patients and limit future diagnosis of skin cancer through primary prevention, the value of the early diagnosis and management of skin cancer cannot be understated. It has the potential to be lifesaving, by giving the physician the opportunity to cure most malignancies with prompt surgical excision. Unfortunately, not all skin cancers are diagnosed early before they affect quality of life and become disfiguring or potentially lethal.

The diagnosis of both non-melanoma skin cancer and melanoma has traditionally been made by inspection and biopsy of suspicious lesions with subsequent histological examination. Clinical diagnosis of melanoma has evolved significantly in the past 40 years. Prior to 1985, melanoma was rarely diagnosed before gross clinical features were present. In 1985, in a joint national program from the American Academy of Dermatology and the American Cancer Society, the ABCD criteria were introduced, which taught many of the features of early melanoma to physicians and the general public. This initiated a massive education and public health campaign that has aided in the earlier diagnosis of melanoma. Despite patient education efforts and prophylactic screening, all forms of skin cancer are still being diagnosed, even at late stages, at alarming rates. The goal for all clinicians should be to strive to increase their ability to detect skin cancer early when it can be effectively treated.

Timely diagnosis of cutaneous malignancy is critical in reducing morbidity, mortality, and the increased health care costs associated with treatment of advanced disease. Despite increasing incidences of all types of skin cancers, detection is now happening earlier before disease becomes disfiguring or advanced. The cornerstone of diagnosis for skin cancers largely remains clinical and continues to evolve with improved recognition and description of common malignant features. Despite advances, unaided visual examination of the skin alone may still be suboptimal in screening for skin cancer. In order to continue to improve early detection and outcomes, the development of accurate, sensitive, and objective diagnostic instruments to help aid the visual diagnosis is important. Technologies are emerging to aid in biopsy decisions, specimen evaluation, and risk stratification, which have the potential to have a tremendous impact on public health and patient outcomes.

This issue of *Dermatologic Clinics* provides a comprehensive overview of the current state of skin cancer diagnosis, the new and emerging technologies within the field, and their integration into daily clinical practice. It is hoped the information presented here will help the readers improve their knowledge related to these issues, helping to reach the goals of attaining earlier detection, decreasing

Dermatol Clin 35 (2017) xv–xvi
http://dx.doi.org/10.1016/j.det.2017.06.019
0733-8635/17/© 2017 Published by Elsevier Inc.

derm.theclinics.com

the number of unnecessary biopsies, improving diagnostic and prognostic accuracy, and reducing costs to both patients and the health care system.

Aaron S. Farberg, MD
Department of Dermatology
Icahn School of Medicine at Mount Sinai
5 East 98th Street Floor 5
New York, NY 10029, USA

Darrell S. Rigel, MD, MS
Department of Dermatology
NYU School of Medicine
35 East 35th Street Suite 208
New York, NY 10016, USA

*E-mail addresses:*
aaron.farberg@gmail.com (A.S. Farberg)
darrell.rigel@gmail.com (D.S. Rigel)

# Clinical Diagnosis of Skin Cancer
## Enhancing Inspection and Early Recognition

Alex M. Glazer, MD[a],*, Darrell S. Rigel, MD, MS[b],
Richard R. Winkelmann, DO[c], Aaron S. Farberg, MD[d]

## KEYWORDS

• Skin cancer • Melanoma • Screening • Detection • Diagnosis • ABCDE

## KEY POINTS

• Early recognition and removal of melanoma and other skin cancers can help prevent significant morbidity and cancer-related deaths and is associated with increased survival.
• Numerous public health initiatives have been used to create awareness of the dangers of skin cancer and to help patients recognize suspicious lesions on themselves.
• Despite technological advancements, the cornerstone of diagnosis of skin cancer remains based on clinical recognition.

## INTRODUCTION

Nonmelanoma (NMSC) and melanoma skin cancer are two of the most commonly diagnosed forms of human malignancy in the United States and worldwide.[1,2] NMSC is far more common but melanoma has a greater lethal potential. Cutaneous malignancy can cause significant morbidity and mortality and has an increased cost of therapy associated with advanced disease. Over the past century, the incidence of skin cancer has increased significantly. However, detection is happening earlier while prognosis is more favorable before disease becomes disfiguring or advanced. For all of these reasons, accurate and effective early clinical diagnosis of skin cancer continues to be paramount.

Over time, approaches for diagnosing NMSC have remained constant based on clinical inspection and patient history of any suspicious lesions that may be growing or changing. The diagnosis of melanoma has evolved significantly over the past century and now more melanomas are being detected at earlier stages. Clinical inspection and recognition of melanoma and NMSC continues to be the cornerstone of diagnosis and management for these cancers.

## CONTENT

The clinical recognition of skin cancer has long been the foundation of identification and diagnosis of malignant skin lesions. Clinical diagnosis of NMSC has been unchanged over the past century. Typically, through patient history, lesions that are red, raised, topographically abnormal, growing, bleeding, crusting, or changing are identified and visually examined. Based on clinical expertise, a decision is made to biopsy and/or treat the suspicious lesions. New technologies now exist that are used in conjunction to increase the accuracy of clinical diagnosis

Disclosure Statement: There are no relevant conflicts of interest to disclose.
[a] Division of Dermatology, Department of Medicine, University of Arizona College of Medicine - Tucson, 1601 N. Campbell Avenue, Tucson, AZ 85719, USA; [b] Clinical Professor, Department of Dermatology, NYU School of Medicine, 35 E 35th Street 208, New York, NY 10016, USA; [c] Department of Dermatology, OhioHealth, 75 Hospital Drive, Suite 250, Athens, OH 45701, USA; [d] Department of Dermatology, Icahn School of Medicine at Mount Sinai, 5 E 98th Street 5th floor, New York, NY 10029, USA
* Corresponding author.
E-mail address: alexglazer@gmail.com

Dermatol Clin 35 (2017) 409–416
http://dx.doi.org/10.1016/j.det.2017.06.001
0733-8635/17/© 2017 Elsevier Inc. All rights reserved.

derm.theclinics.com

(discussed elsewhere in this issue), but few have been widely adopted.

In contrast, diagnosis and treatment of melanoma has evolved significantly since this neoplasm was first recognized as a disease entity more than 200 years ago. The importance of early diagnosis of melanoma cannot be understated. Melanoma first grows horizontally within the epidermis (superficial or horizontal growth phase) and over time penetrates and grows vertically into the dermis (invasive or vertical growth phase).[3] Prognosis is directly proportional to the vertical depth of the neoplasm, so early detection has the potential to significantly limit disease burden and decrease cancer deaths. Most health care costs associated with melanoma occur with treatment of advanced disease demonstrating that there are also significant cost savings associated with earlier detection.[4]

Despite increasing incidence for all histologic subtypes and thicknesses of melanoma, the survival rates have steadily improved.[5] Overall 5-year survival rates for invasive melanoma increased from 82% to 93% from 1979 to 2008.[6] Earlier detection has generally led to a greater proportion of thinner depth lesions being removed, which typically are associated with improved outcomes. For thin lesions, treatment is usually surgical excision without the need for further work-up, which results in significant health care savings.

Although melanoma is now more frequently detected earlier, this has not always been the case. Before the 1980s, melanomas were often not diagnosed until gross clinical signs or metastatic disease was present and prognosis was generally poor. There were few advances that had occurred to improve patient awareness or clinician recognition because the clinical features of early melanoma were not well described. Diagnosis was typically made by inspection for gross clinical features including but not limited to extremely large size, bleeding, ulceration, and fungation. This led to a high disease burden and poor prognosis at the time of diagnosis.

The importance of early detection was first understood in the 1960s. Clark and colleagues[7] first correlated the level of histologic invasion, from the epidermis to the subcutaneous fat, with the likely progression and prognosis of disease. In 1970, Breslow[8] then demonstrated that prognosis was proportional to thickness, depth of invasion, and volume of the primary malignancy. He also noted that metastasis rarely occurred in lesions less than 0.76 mm in thickness. Since 1970 numerous studies have confirmed this concept that thinner lesions directly correlate with increased survival and better prognosis.[9] The

goal of developing guidelines to detect melanoma earlier, when lesions were thinner and had a better prognosis, was therefore imperative to increase overall survival.

Before the 1980s, the clinical characteristics of early melanoma were not well described. Detecting melanoma was typically a learned entity based on many years of clinical experience. There was a critical need to educate less-experienced dermatologists, other physicians, and the general public on features of early melanoma to improve disease outcomes. In 1985, dermatologists at New York University devised the ABCD (Asymmetry, Border irregularity, Color variegation, Diameter >6 mm) acronym to help aid in the clinical diagnosis of early melanoma.[10] This study demonstrated that these parameters were some of the most commonly encountered clinical features seen in early melanomas and served as a guideline for atypical features that should be potentially concerning in pigmented skin lesion (PSL)s.

The ABCDs were intended to help describe and differentiate early, thin melanomas that might be confused with benign PSLs. Its straightforward nature allowed it to be used by clinicians and laypeople to identify potentially suspicious lesions before gross symptoms occurred. Ulcerated and elevated features were excluded because they were suggestive of more advanced disease. In 2004, a fifth parameter was added to the mnemonic, E (Evolving), making it the ABCDE criteria (**Table 1**).[11] The addition of E improved the ability to recognize melanoma earlier because it includes lesions that are changing size, shape, or color and does not preclude lesions less than 6 mm.

Because of the diverse nature of early melanoma, one or more of the ABCDEs may be lacking, especially in early disease. Diameter has been the most controversial parameter, because as early diagnosis has improved, many melanomas less than 6 mm wide are now being identified. However, recent studies have reconfirmed that diameter remains a useful differentiating parameter.[12]

The ABCDE criteria have been verified in multiple studies that have demonstrated their sensitivity, specificity, and diagnostic accuracy.[13–16] The sensitivity and specificity of these parameters when used individually ranges from 57% to 90% and 59% to 90%, respectively.[17] Determining quantitative ABCDs through the use of computer image analysis has reinforced these findings.[18] Sensitivity and specificity both increase when criteria are used in conjunction with one another. Additionally, studies have demonstrated high interrater reliability and objectivity in assessing these clinical features, enhancing their utility as a screening measure.[19]

**Table 1**
**ABCDE tools for detection of early melanoma**

| | Description | Illustration |
|---|---|---|
| Asymmetry | Lesions cannot easily be divided in half so that one half looks like the other. | |
| Border irregularity | Borders are typically not well defined and are irregularly shaped. | |
| Color variegation | One or more colors or variations in color. Colors frequently include black, brown, and tan. Less frequently red, white, or blue may be present. | |
| Diameter | Most early melanomas are >6 mm (approximately the size of a pencil eraser). | |
| Evolving | Lesions that are changing in size, shape, color, topography, sensation, consistency or to the surrounding skin. | |

With the advent of the ABCDEs the level of diagnosis of melanoma improved for dermatologists and nondermatologists.[20] The ABCDE parameters are well known and frequently used by groups including the American Academy of Dermatology and the American Cancer Society. Like any tool, the ABCDEs have strengths and limitations (ie, may not be as effective in recognizing early nodular melanoma), but for now they remain a valuable component of the early detection campaign against melanoma.[21]

In addition to the ABCDEs, other clinical diagnostic paradigms have been developed to enhance the early recognition and diagnosis of melanoma. The revised Glasgow seven-point checklist includes three major criteria (change in size/new lesion, change in shape, change in color) and four minor criteria (diameter >7 mm, inflammation, crusting or bleeding, and sensory changes)

(Table 2).[22] The presence of any of the major criteria is an indication for a referral and the additional presence of any minor criteria reinforces the need for referral. One study evaluating the

**Table 2**
**Revised Glasgow 7-point checklist**

| Major Features[a] | Minor Features[b] |
|---|---|
| Change in lesion size | Inflammation |
| | Itch or altered sensation |
| Irregular pigmentation | Larger than other lesions (diameter >7 mm) |
| Irregular border | Oozing/crusting of lesion |

[a] Presence of any of the major features is an indication for a referral.
[b] Additional presence of any minor features reaffirms the need for referral.

sensitivity and specificity of the Glasgow checklist found a sensitivity of 100% and a specificity of 37% for 165 evaluated lesions.[23] Other studies of only melanomas have demonstrated higher specificity.[24] The Glasgow checklist has been less widely adopted than the ABCDEs, likely because of its greater complexity with similar efficacy in identifying concerning PSLs.

The "ugly duckling" sign is another commonly used clinical diagnostic tool to recognize lesions suspicious for melanoma. This is based on the assumption that patients with many nevi tend to have normal nevi that resemble one another morphologically[25] or signature nevi.[26] This concept implies that a PSL that looks morphologically different from the signature nevi of a patient should be considered suspicious, even if it does not fulfill the ABCDE or seven-point criteria. Although the predictive value of the ugly duckling sign has not been systematically evaluated, it

has been shown to be sensitive for dermatologists and nondermatologists.[27]

Routine self-skin examination (SSE) is another tool that reinforces the educational experience that patients have beyond their physician-driven total body skin examination. Monthly SSE can alert patients to any new or changing lesions, which can be brought to the attention of their dermatologist for further evaluation to enhance early recognition (**Figs. 1–3**). SSE may be associated with a reduced risk of melanoma-associated mortality.[10,28] Although the efficacy of SSE is still debated, it is a free, noninvasive, and nondangerous method that allows the patient to serve as a partner for their early detection efforts.

Other less commonly known diagnostic parameters for clinically identifying melanoma exist. The CUBED (Colored lesions different from skin color, *U*ncertain diagnosis, *B*leeding lesions, *E*nlarging lesions despite therapy, *D*elay in healing beyond

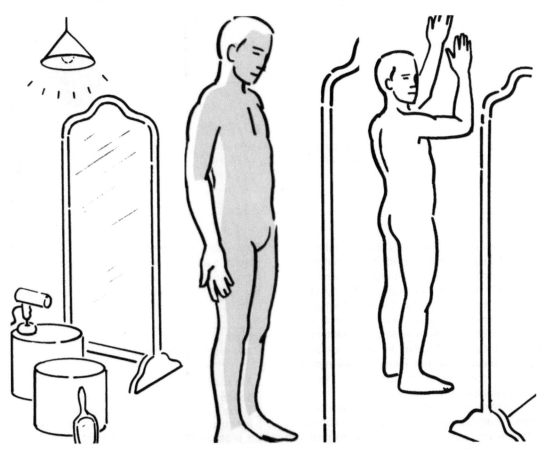

**Fig. 1.** Self-examination equipment includes a full-length mirror, a handheld mirror, a blow dryer, and two stools in a well-lit room. The front of the body should be inspected in a full-length mirror. Then the sides should be examined by turning to one side and raising your arms with the palms. (*From* Friedman RJ, Rigel DS, Kopf AW. Early detection of malignant melanoma: the role of physician examination and self-examination of the skin. CA Cancer J Clin 1985;35:146–9; with permission.)

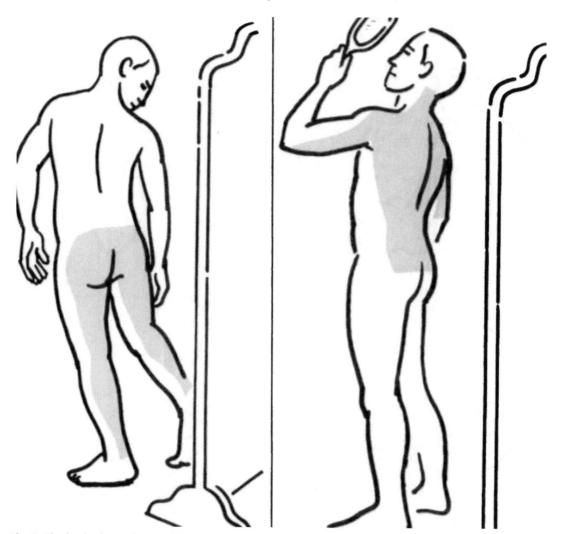

**Fig. 2.** The back of your legs and buttocks should be examined in a full-length mirror. The handheld mirror is used with your back facing the full-length mirror to examine the back of the neck, back, and scalp. (*From* Friedman RJ, Rigel DS, Kopf AW. Early detection of malignant melanoma: the role of physician examination and self-examination of the skin. CA Cancer J Clin 1985;35:146–9; with permission.)

2 months) criteria were developed to help diagnose melanoma of the foot and nail. If any two of the characteristics are present, it is an indication for referral for evaluation of the suspicious lesion.[29] In addition, many authors have attempted to modify the ABCDEs with the addition of other characteristics in hopes of increasing diagnostic accuracy, but none of these iterations have been proven to be superior or widely adopted.[21]

These systematic approaches for the evaluation of PSLs have helped dermatologists and lay people improve their ability to clinically recognize early melanoma. Although none of the previously mentioned methods are perfect, they provide simple guidelines that are used by dermatologists,

general practitioners, and lay people to recognize warning signs of early melanoma.

Because of its diverse nature, clinical recognition of melanoma is challenging even for experienced dermatologists. To make the clinical diagnosis of melanoma, one must have a high index of suspicion. A thorough knowledge of clinical features of melanoma, characteristics of different variants of melanoma, and the clinical features of other PSLs that need to be differentiated from melanoma is imperative. Additionally, knowledge of factors associated with increased risk of developing melanoma including family or personal history of melanoma, presence of many nevi, sunburn history, and fair skin types must also be taken into account.

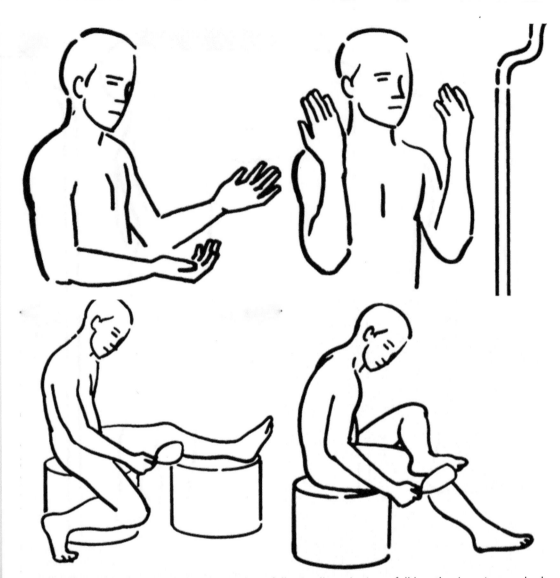

**Fig. 3.** The hands and arms should be inspected carefully visually and using a full-length mirror. Legs and soles should be examined one leg at a time using a handheld mirror to visualize the entire surface area. (*From* Friedman RJ, Rigel DS, Kopf AW. Early detection of malignant melanoma: the role of physician examination and self-examination of the skin. CA Cancer J Clin 1985;35:146–9; with permission.)

The actual sensitivity for diagnosis of early melanoma in the clinical setting is difficult to assess. The biopsy ratio (the proportion of melanoma to total number of biopsied PSLs) is not a useful parameter because, in the case of a potentially lethal malignancy, erring on the side of overbiopsying carries less risk than underbiopsying leading to missed cancer. The best way to assess accuracy is through reader studies where dermatologists are given images of biopsy-confirmed lesions and asked to provide a presumptive diagnosis. Several reader studies have shown sensitivities between 71% and 82% for dermatologists at

identifying early melanoma based on their decision to biopsy depending on appearance alone.[30,31] Greater sensitivities are achieved in clinical practice in specialized pigmented lesion centers.[32]

New technologies have been developed that can help further improve the accuracy of skin cancer beyond clinical inspection alone. These include whole-body photography, dermoscopy, reflectance confocal microscopy, optical coherence tomography, multispectral imaging and analysis, and smartphone-based applications (all discussed elsewhere in this issue). Despite these advances in technology, it continues to take a trained dermatologist and a good set of eyes to help identify which lesions are suspicious and should be screened to use these technologies most efficiently.[33]

Other public health measures are now being used to promote earlier clinical detection of NMSC and melanoma. Patient education initiatives with descriptions of concerning lesions and instructions for home SSEs can help improve patients' ability to detect suspicious lesions. Annual physician-driven total body skin examinations can help to recognize and remove suspicious lesions. More frequent physician examinations are useful in high-risk patients who have personal history of skin malignancy, family history of melanoma, history of high number of nevi, or personal or family history of dysplastic nevi. Mass skin screening programs have also been undertaken by the American Academy of Dermatology and various other volunteer groups to enhance secondary prevention and to provide a teachable moment to educate patients on skin cancer.

## SUMMARY

Despite the many technological advancements occurring in skin cancer diagnosis, visual evaluation continues to be paramount in this process. The clinical evaluation of melanoma has been significantly refined over the past 30 years. Although guidelines have helped clinicians become more familiar with the features of melanoma, it still takes a high index of suspicion and thorough knowledge of the patient's history to most efficiently diagnose skin cancer.

Neville Davis[34] once said "unlike other cancers, which are generally hidden from view, malignant melanoma writes its message in the skin with its own ink and it is there for all of us to see. Some see, but do not comprehend." The same holds true for NMSC. Even though cutaneous malignancy is in plain sight, many people cannot readily recognize it. Over the past half century, clinical diagnosis of melanoma and survival rates of skin cancers have improved steadily as a function of patient education and public health initiatives. Although clinical examination will continue to be augmented by new technologies that allow physicians to better "comprehend" what they are seeing, technology will never be able to supersede an experienced clinician with a good set of eyes to choose the proper lesions to screen.

## REFERENCES

1. Rogers HW, Weinstock MA, Feldman SR, et al. Incidence estimate of nonmelanoma skin cancer (keratinocyte carcinomas) in US population, 2012. JAMA Dermatol 2015;151(10):1081–6.
2. Tripp MK, Watson M, Balk SJ, et al. State of the science on prevention and screening to reduce melanoma incidence and mortality: the time is now. CA Cancer J Clin 2016. http://dx.doi.org/10.3322/caac.21352.
3. Clark WH Jr, Elder DE, Guerry D 4th, et al. Model predicting survival in stage I melanoma based on tumor progression. J Natl Cancer Inst 1989;81(24):1893–904.
4. Tsao H, Rogers GS, Sober AJ. An estimate of the annual direct cost of treating cutaneous melanoma. J Am Acad Dermatol 1998;38(5 Pt 1):669–80.
5. Linos E, Swetter SM, Cockburn MG, et al. Increasing burden of melanoma in the United States. J Invest Dermatol 2009;129(7):1666–74.
6. Siegel R, Naishadham D, Jemal A. Cancer statistics, 2013. CA Cancer J Clin 2013;63:11–30.
7. Clark WH Jr, From L, Bernardino EA, et al. The histiogenesis and biologic behavior or primary human malignant melanomas of the skin. Cancer Res 1969;29(3):705–27.
8. Breslow A. Thickness, cross sectional area and depth of invasion in prognosis of cutaneous melanoma. Ann Surg 1970;174:902–8.
9. Balch CM, Soong SJ, Gershenwald JE, et al. Prognostic factors analysis of 17,600 melanoma patients: validation of the American Joint Committee on Cancer melanoma staging system. J Clin Oncol 2001;19:3622–34.
10. Friedman RJ, Rigel DS, Kopf AW. Early detection of malignant melanoma: the role of physician examination and self-examination of the skin. CA Cancer J Clin 1985;35:130–51.
11. Abbasi NR, Shaw HM, Rigel DS, et al. Early diagnosis of cutaneous melanoma: revisiting the ABCD criteria. JAMA 2004;292(22):2771–6.
12. Abbasi NR, Yancovitz M, Gutkowicz-Krusin D, et al. Utility of lesion diameter in the clinical diagnosis of cutaneous melanoma. Arch Dermatol 2008;144(4):469–74.
13. Carli P, De Giorgi V, Crocetti E, et al. Diagnostic and referral accuracy of family doctors in melanoma screening: effect of a short formal training. Eur J Cancer Prev 2005;14:51–5.
14. Peuvrel L, Quereux G, Jumbou B, et al. Impact of a campaign to train general practitioners in screening for melanoma. Eur J Cancer Prev 2009;18:225–9.
15. Betti R, Vergani R, Tolomio E. Factors of delay in the diagnosis of melanoma. Eur J Dermatol 2003;14:183–8.
16. Branstrom R, Hedblad MA, Krakau I, et al. Laypersons' perceptual discrimination of pigmented skin lesions. J Am Acad Dermatol 2002;46:667–73.
17. Thomas L, Tranchand P, Berard F, et al. Semiological value of ABCDE criteria in the diagnosis of

cutaneous pigmented tumors. Dermatology 1998;
197(1):11–7.

18. Glazer AM, Winkelmann RR, Farberg AS, et al.
Quantitative ABCD parameters measured by a multispectral digital skin lesion analysis device for evaluation of suspicious pigmented lesions strongly
correlate with clinical ABCD observations. J Am
Acad Dermatol 2017;76(6):AB212(Suppl 1).

19. Barnhill RL, Roush GC, Ernstoff MS, et al. Interclini-
cian agreement on the recognition of selected gross
morphologic features of pigmented lesions. Studies
of melanocytic nevi V. J Am Acad Dermatol 1992;26:
185–90.

20. Whited JD, Grichnik JM. Does this patient have a
mole or a melanoma? JAMA 1998;279:696–701.

21. Tsao H, Olazagasti JM, Cordoro KM, et al. Early
detection of melanoma: reviewing the ABCDEs.
J Am Acad Dermatol 2015;72(4):717–23.

22. Mackie RM. Clinical recognition of early invasive malignant melanoma. BMJ 1990;134:103–4.

23. Healsmith MF, Bourke JF, Osborne JE, et al. An evaluation of the revised seven-point checklist for the
early diagnosis of cutaneous malignant melanoma.
Br J Dermatol 1994;130(1):48.

24. du Vivier AW, Williams HC, Brett JV, et al. How do
malignant melanomas present and does this correlate with the seven-point checklist? Clin Exp Dermatol 1991;16(5):344.

25. Grob JJ, Bonerandi JJ. The "ugly duckling" sign:
identification of the common characteristics of nevi
in an individual as a basis for melanoma screening.
Arch Dermatol 1998;134(1):103–4.

26. Suh KT, Bolognia JL. Signature nevi. J Am Acad Dermatol 2009;60(3):508–14.

27. Scope A, Dusza SW, Halpern AC, et al. The "ugly
duckling" sign: agreement between observers.
Arch Dermatol 2008;144(1):58–64.

28. Berwick M, Begg CB, Fine JA, et al. Screening for
cutaneous melanoma by skin self-examination.
J Natl Cancer Inst 1996;88(1):17–23.

29. Bristow IR, de Berker DA, Acland KM, et al. Clinical
guidelines for the recognition of melanoma of the
foot and nail unit. J Foot Ankle Res 2010;3:25.

30. Rigel DS, Roy M, Yoo J, et al. Impact guidance from
computer-aided multispectral digital skin lesion
analysis device on decision to biopsy lesions clinically suggestive of melanoma. Arch Dermatol
2012;148(4):541–3.

31. Friedman RJ, Gutkowicz-Krusin D, Farber MJ, et al.
The diagnostic performance of expert dermoscopists vs a computer-vision system on small-diameter
melanomas. Arch Dermatol 2008;144:476–82.

32. Carli P, Nardini P, Crocetti E, et al. Frequency and
characteristics of melanomas missed at a pigmented lesion clinic: a registry-based study. Melanoma Res 2004;14(5):403–7.

33. Dreiseitl S, Binder M, Hable K, et al. Computer
versus human diagnosis of melanoma: evaluation
of the feasibility of an automated diagnostic system
in a prospective clinical trial. Melanoma Res 2009;
19(3):180–4.

34. Davis N. Modern concepts of melanoma and its
management. Ann Plast Surg 1978;1:628–30.

# Enhancing Skin Cancer Diagnosis with Dermoscopy

Zachary J. Wolner, BA, Oriol Yélamos, MD,
Konstantinos Liopyris, MD, Tova Rogers, MFA,
Michael A. Marchetti, MD, Ashfaq A. Marghoob, MD*

## KEYWORDS

- Dermoscopy • Dermatoscopy • Keratinocyte carcinomas • Diagnostic accuracy • Sensitivity
- Specificity • Odds ratio • Melanoma

## KEY POINTS

- Dermoscopy increases diagnostic accuracy and sensitivity for melanoma, and helps in the detection of thinner tumors.
- Multiple studies have established that dermoscopy is an aid for diagnosing basal cell carcinoma; the presence of dermoscopic criteria can predict the histopathological subtype of basal cell carcinoma.
- Although actinic keratosis, Bowen disease/squamous cell carcinoma in situ, invasive squamous cell carcinoma, and keratoacanthoma share common dermoscopic features, specific criteria can permit diagnostic discrimination.
- Dermoscopy novices can benefit from using diagnostic or triage algorithms to improve their diagnostic abilities and management decisions.

## INTRODUCTION

Dermoscopy has been shown to increase sensitivity for skin cancer detection, decrease the benign-to-malignant biopsy ratio, and allow for the diagnosis of thinner melanomas compared with naked eye examination (NEE).[1–3] In 2009, a survey of academic dermatologists and chief residents in US dermatology training programs demonstrated that 84% of attending dermatologists used dermoscopy in daily practice and 90.2% of chief dermatology residents received dermoscopy training as part of their curricula.[4] These findings represented a significant increase in training and use of dermoscopy compared with a similar survey performed 10 years before.[5] The use of dermoscopy has also increased among nondermatologist physicians who actively participate in skin cancer management, such as family physicians.[6–8]

Despite the growing number of practitioners incorporating dermoscopy into their daily practices, there remain significant barriers, such as lack of training resources, preventing its widespread adoption.[4] Dermoscopic teaching methodologies, which include pattern analysis, diagnostic algorithms, and simplified triage algorithms, continue to emerge.

Funding: This research was funded in part through the NIH/NCI Cancer Center Support Grant P30 CA008748.
Conflict of Interest: The authors have no conflicts of interest to declare.
Permissions: Natalia Jaimes, MD has granted permission to use select schematics throughout this article. Natalia Jaimes, MD and the coauthors retain the copyright to any line drawing included in this submission.
Dermatology Service, Department of Medicine, Memorial Sloan Kettering Cancer Center, 16 East 60th Street, New York, NY 10022, USA
* Corresponding author.
E-mail address: marghooa@mskcc.org

Dermatol Clin 35 (2017) 417–437
http://dx.doi.org/10.1016/j.det.2017.06.003
0733-8635/17/© 2017 Elsevier Inc. All rights reserved.

They aim to provide an entry point in educating beginners in dermoscopy. Here, the authors review the diagnostic utility of dermoscopy for detection of melanoma and keratinocyte carcinomas (KC; also known as nonmelanoma skin cancers) and outline the specific dermoscopic features that can help discriminate these cancers from benign lesions. A review of dermoscopic teaching methodologies, including triage algorithms, is also provided.

## DERMOSCOPY FOR THE DIAGNOSIS AND MANAGEMENT OF CUTANEOUS MELANOMA

In 2001, the first meta-analysis of the diagnostic power of dermoscopy found dermoscopy to be more accurate than NEE alone for the diagnosis of cutaneous melanoma.[9] Two additional meta-analyses have since reinforced these findings.[2,10] The most recent, by Vestergaard and colleagues,[2] included only prospective studies performed in a clinical setting and thus more accurately reflected everyday dermoscopy use. In total, 8487 suspicious pigmented and nonpigmented lesions were included, and melanoma prevalence ranged from 0.5% to 21.1% with a Breslow thickness that ranged from 0.35 to 0.95 mm.[2] Dermoscopic and clinical accuracy were evaluated through the diagnostic odds ratio (DOR), which considers both sensitivity and specificity and their respective tradeoffs.[2] The DOR for dermoscopy was 15.6 (confidence interval [CI]: 2.9–83.7, $P = .016$) times higher for dermoscopy than NEE. A summary estimate of sensitivity was higher with dermoscopy (0.90, CI: 0.80–0.95) than for NEE (0.71, CI: 0.59–82, $P = .002$)[2]; although specificity was higher for dermoscopy (0.90, CI: 0.57–98) than NEE (0.81, CI: 0.48–0.95, $P = .18$), it was not statistically significant.[2]

In all 3 meta-analyses, diagnostic accuracy was dependent upon the experience of the examiner.[2,9,10] However, inexperienced users, after a 2-hour course, had an improved sensitivity without compromising their specificity.[2] Terushkin and colleagues[11] found, through assessment of the benign-to-malignant biopsy ratio (BMR), that a single dermatologist newly adopting dermoscopy experienced a learning curve. Initially, the BMR of the dermatologist increased compared with NEE, but with time and experience, the BMR dropped below the baseline value with NEE alone and approached the level of pigmented lesion specialists. Several studies have demonstrated that short training modules can improve the diagnostic performance of inexperienced dermatologists, general practitioners, and even medical students.[6,12,13] However, the training modalities

have varied widely among studies, and the ideal teaching method for beginners remains to be standardized.

The BMR (which is directly related to positive predictive value), although not a surrogate, is impacted by the sensitivity and specificity of dermoscopy. Improvements in this ratio suggest that the increased sensitivity seen with dermoscopy does not entail an increase in the number of unnecessary biopsies and thus an increase in morbidity. Carli and colleagues[1] retrospectively examined 2 users before and after the introduction of dermoscopy and 4 nonusers. Analysis demonstrated a significant improvement in the BMR over a 4-year study period in the dermoscopy arm (18:1–4.3:1, $P = .037$). The BMR for nonusers had no significant difference at the beginning and the end of the study (11.8:1–14.8:1).[1] In a randomized controlled trial comparing one-time evaluations of equivocal pigmented lesions with dermoscopy or NEE, 9% of patients followed with dermoscopy were referred for biopsy or excision compared with 15.6% with NEE ($P = .013$). The reduction in surgical morbidity was not hindered by a decreased ability to diagnose melanoma.[14] Finally, a multicenter survey over 10 years showed that the BMR at sites dedicated to skin cancer treatment improved from 12.8 to 6.8 ($P<.001$) and remained unchanged in sites not dedicated to screening for skin cancer. The investigators of that study argue that the introduction of dermoscopy was largely responsible for the observed improvement in the BMR.[15]

Dermoscopy and dermoscopic screening allow for the earlier detection of melanoma and improved clinical management. Several studies have shown that dermoscopic monitoring of lesions enables the detection of thin, featureless melanomas.[3,16] In a meta-analysis with a mean follow-up of 30 months, Salerni and colleagues[3] showed dermoscopy users to detect a greater number of thinner melanomas compared with NEE (mean Breslow depth 0.77 mm vs 1.43 mm, $P<.05$). Haenssle and colleagues[16] found that participation in specialized dermoscopic screening programs and dermoscopic examinations at the time of diagnosis were also significantly associated with thinner melanomas ($P<.01$). Dermoscopy users have identified melanoma-specific dermoscopic features that have enabled them to recognize melanoma with the sensitivity and specificity described. The following sections expand upon these melanoma-specific dermoscopic features and other features for basal cell carcinoma (BCC) and keratinizing carcinomas.

## DERMOSCOPIC FEATURES IN MELANOMA

By allowing for the in vivo assessment of subsurface skin structures, dermoscopy offers a window into the histologic diagnosis of skin cancers.[17] Many of the described dermoscopic features have known histologic correlates. The presence of these features can provide insight into the cellular nature of skin neoplasms and allow for more precise clinical diagnoses. When the dermoscopic diagnosis is unclear, structures can hint at malignant potential. Although the dermoscopic features discussed in **Table 1** can be applied to any lesion on the skin, there are additional criteria in **Table 2** that are specific to lesions on the face, mucosa, nails, and volar surfaces, which are outlined in later discussion. Examples of dermoscopic features found in melanoma are shown in **Fig. 1**.

Lentigo maligna and lentigo maligna melanoma both arise on sun-damaged skin, most commonly the face and scalp (both lentigo maligna and lentigo maligna melanoma are represented by the abbreviation LMM). The anatomic predilection for the face and sun-damaged skin entails a broad differential diagnosis, including pigmented actinic keratosis (AK), lichen planus-like keratoses, and early-flat seborrheic keratoses.[18] Dermoscopy can help the user sort through the numerous diagnoses. Facial skin has a flattened dermoepidermal junction resulting in absence of traditional reticular patterns commonly seen in melanocytic lesions. Instead, the pigmentation is punctuated by adnexal structures, creating a pseudonetwork.[19] LMM-specific structures include asymmetrical pigmentation of follicular openings, dots aggregated around adnexal openings, polygonal lines and rhomboid structures, and dark blotches with or without obliteration of the adnexal openings (**Fig. 2**A).[18,20,21]

Additional dermoscopic features are also needed to evaluate for melanoma arising on the nail apparatus, mucosa, or volar skin. In melanoma of the nail apparatus, dermoscopy of the pigmented band will show multiple brown to black lines with irregular arrangement and thickness and possible areas of pigment interruption (see **Fig. 2**B).[22] The mucosa comprises a wide range of anatomic sites, such as the lip, glans penis, anogenital orifice, labia, and praeputium. On dermoscopy, an early sign of mucosal melanoma is the presence of structureless areas and gray color. More advanced melanoma can present with multiple patterns and colors, particularly white, blue, and/or gray (see **Fig. 2**C).[23,24] The dermoscopic appearance of acral lentiginous melanoma (ALM) is shaped by the unique furrow and ridge pattern of acral volar skin surfaces. Melanocytic features specific to ALM are the parallel ridge pattern and irregular diffuse pigmentation (see **Fig. 2**D).[25] **Tables 1** and **2** provide an overview of melanoma-specific criteria, including definitions, pictorial examples, and reported sensitivities, specificities, and odds ratios. This list was compiled using the most recent definitions of dermoscopic criteria published by the International Dermoscopy Society in 2016.[27]

## DERMOSCOPY FOR THE DIAGNOSIS AND MANAGEMENT OF KERATINOCYTE CARCINOMAS

In addition to differentiating nevi from melanoma and detecting early melanoma, dermoscopy can also be used to detect KC. Rosendahl and colleagues[28] examined 217 consecutive pigmented nonmelanocytic lesions, of which 138 were malignant, with both dermoscopy and NEE. They reported a diagnostic improvement with dermoscopy of 0.89 (area under the receiver operating curve) compared with 0.83 with NEE alone ($P<.001$). In a 2016, 2-part study of optional then mandatory dermoscopy use, the overall diagnostic sensitivity of BCC was 93.3% (91.9–94.5) and specificity was 91.8% (90.6–93.0).[29] Furthermore, dermoscopy when compared with NEE was shown to help predict BCC histopathology subtypes.[29] In the following sections, the specific diagnostic features of KC are detailed further.

## DERMOSCOPIC FEATURES IN BASAL CELL CARCINOMA

BCCs are broadly classified as pigmented or nonpigmented. Although most BCCs on NEE are nonpigmented, 29.8% of these lesions actually reveal pigment structures when viewed with dermoscopy.[30] The pigmented structures seen in BCC include blue-gray globules or ovoid nests, spoke-wheel structures, and leaflike areas. The structures seen in nonpigmented or pigmented BCC include arborizing vessels, shiny white blotches and strands (seen with polarized dermoscopy), and ulcers/erosions (**Table 3**).[31–33] Studies have demonstrated that certain dermoscopic structures and patterns are associated with different subtypes of BCC.[29,34] The presence of spoke-wheel and leaflike structures, multiple small erosions, short fine vessels, and shiny white blotches and strands in a nonpalpable lesion is associated with superficial BCC. In contrast, the presence of blue-gray globules, ovoid nest, arborizing vessels, and ulceration is associated with nodular BCC.[29,34] Examples of dermoscopic features found in BCC are shown in **Fig. 3**.

**Table 1**
Dermoscopic features of melanoma

| Dermoscopic Structures | Schematic Illustration | Definition/Significance | Diagnostic Value | |
|---|---|---|---|---|
| Atypical pigment network and angulated lines | | Atypical pigment network has a disorganized and asymmetric distribution, areas of disruption, and/or significant variability in line thickness and color. In addition, the holes of the network are of differing sizes and shapes. An atypical network can appear "out of focus" with smudging of the network lines and/or with gray color.[27] An atypical network is associated with superficial spreading melanoma[56] | Sensitivity | 21%[57]; 52%–77.1%[58–61]; 100%[62] |
| | | Angulated lines create a zigzag pattern with lines merging to create polygonal structures such as rhomboids. Angulated lines usually have a gray color and are associated with melanoma on sun-damaged skin, which includes lentigo maligna and lentigo maligna melanoma[31] | Specificity | 46%[62]; 64.7%–88.5%[57–61,63] |
| | | | Odds ratio | 2.0–2.8[18,44,57,61]; 9[39] |
| Negative network | | Negative network consists of elongated and curvilinear globular structures that are surrounded by hypopigmentation. The hypopigmentation takes on the appearance of serpiginous lines meandering between the hyperpigmented elongated structures.[27] A negative network is associated with melanomas arising in nevi[64] | Sensitivity | 22% – 34.6%[54,62] |
| | | | Specificity | 77.2%–95%[54,62] |
| | | | Odds ratio | 1.4[44]; 1.8[54] |
| Atypical dots/globules | | Dots and globules consist of round to oval structures of differing size, color, and distribution. In melanoma, the dots tend to be black-brown in color, are not located on the lines of the network, and are distributed in a disorganized fashion. Globules in melanoma tend to vary in color from blue-black to brown, have increased variability in size and shape, and are distributed in a disorganized manner[27] | Sensitivity | 13%–39.6%[57,58,60,61] |
| | | | Specificity | 74.3%–92%[57,58,60,61] |
| | | | Odds ratio | 1.7–4.8[39,57,58] |

| | | | |
|---|---|---|---|
| Irregular streaks | | Streaks, which encompass *pseudopods and radial streaming*, are linear projections located at the perimeter of the lesion that radiate from the tumor toward normal skin[27] | Sensitivity 4.8%–23%[57,60–62] 32%[58]; 58%[59] |
| | | *Pseudopods* are linear projections with small knobs at their tips. *Radial streaming* are the same structures without the knobs. Streaks are a manifestation of radial growth and are associated with superficial spreading melanoma, especially when distributed focally at the periphery.[27,62] Pseudopods appear to have a higher odds ratio than streaming[44] | Specificity 62%[59]; 77%[58]; 90.2%–98.7%[57,60–63] Odds ratio 1.5–5.8[39,44,57,58,61] |
| Regression structures | | Regression structures consist of nonpalpable areas revealing peppering/granularity and scarlike depigmentation. Peppering/granularity and scarlike depigmentation often occur together but can also present independently *Peppering/granularity* consists of fine to coarse dots with a blue-gray color. *Scar-like depigmentation* consists of white areas that are lighter in color than the adjacent normal skin.[27] In areas of scarlike depigmentation, one will not see shiny white lines/ crystalline structures or blood vessels | Sensitivity 11.4%–41.7%[57,58,60–62]; 79%[59] Specificity 63%[59]; 83.5%–99%[57,58,60–62] Odds ratio 2–5.7[39,44,61]; 18.3[58] |
| Blue-white veil | | *Blue-white veil* consists of palpable areas having a blue-black color with an overlying whitish ground-glass haze.[27] The blue white veil corresponds with melanin/melanocytes in the dermis in association with compact orthokeratosis[65] | Sensitivity 11.4%–28%[57,60,61]; 51[62]; 92%[59] Specificity 74%–99.0%[57,59–63] Odds ratio 1.74–2.5[44,58,61]; 13[39] |

(continued on next page)

**Table 1**
*(continued)*

| Dermoscopic Structures | Schematic Illustration | Definition/Significance | Diagnostic Value | |
|---|---|---|---|---|
| Shiny white lines | | *Shiny white lines* (formerly known as *crystalline structures*) are only visible under polarized light and consist of short bright white line(s) that, when in groups, often have a parallel or orthogonal orientation to each other. The presence of these structures is suggestive of melanoma or Spitz nevus and when present in melanoma are associated with invasion[53,62] | Sensitivity | 70.0%[53] |
| | | | Specificity | 80.6%[53] |
| | | | Odds ratio | 2.5[44]; 9.7[53] |
| Atypical blotch | | *Blotches* are an area of heavy pigmentation that obscures the ability to see any other structures in that area. *Atypical or irregular blotches* are defined as the presence of more than one blotch or the presence of an off center blotch located toward the periphery of the lesion[27] | Sensitivity | 18%–37.5%[57,58,60]; 71.3%[61] |
| | | | Specificity | 30.5%[61]; 88.2%–92.6%[57,58,60] |
| | | | Odds ratio | 1.88–4.1[39,44,57,61] |
| Polymorphous vessels | | *Polymorphous vessels* are defined as multiple types of vessels in a single lesion.[27] Except for comma-shaped vessels seen in intradermal nevi, any vessel or vascular blush (milky red areas) seen in a melanocytic lesion should raise concern for melanoma. Melanomas can reveal dotted vessels, serpentine vessels, tortuous vessels, and milky red areas. The vascular structures with the strongest association with melanoma include multiple shades of pink and/or polymorphous vessels. The most predictive vasculature for melanoma is the combination of dotted and serpentine vessels[57] | Sensitivity | 9.4%[60]; 18%[61]; 62.9%[57] |
| | | | Specificity | 53.8%[57]; 91.2%[61]; 96.1%[60] |
| | | | Odds ratio | 2.0–3.04[44,57,61] |

*Courtesy of Natalia Jaimes, MD, Miami, FL.*

**Table 2**
**Dermoscopic features of melanoma arising in special locations**

| | Dermoscopic Structures | Schematic Illustration | Definition/Significance | Diagnostic Value |
|---|---|---|---|---|
| Melanoma of the face | Blotches with obliteration of follicles | | *Blotches with obliteration of follicles* are defined by the loss of visible adnexal openings forming the pseudonetwork typically seen in facial melanocytic tumors.[21] Blotches may be present with preservation of the follicle | Sensitivity — <br> Specificity — <br> Odds ratio 3.82[21] |
| | Concentric circles | | *Concentric circles* (also known as circles within circles) are pigmented rings each surrounding an additional circle.[44] The pigmented ring can be seen within the adnexal opening | Sensitivity 4.2%[18] <br> Specificity 98.8%[18] <br> Odds ratio 2.0[18] |
| | Gray circles | | *Gray circles* are small rings that appear within follicular openings[21] | Sensitivity 54.2%[18] <br> Specificity 83.3%[18] <br> Odds ratio 2.86[21], 4.6[18] |

*(continued on next page)*

**Table 2**
*(continued)*

| Dermoscopic Structures | Schematic Illustration | Definition/Significance | Diagnostic Value |
|---|---|---|---|
| Asymmetric follicular opening (incomplete circles) | | *Asymmetric follicular openings (incomplete circles) are* pigment rings that do not uniformly surround an adnexal opening[27] | Sensitivity 58.3%[18]<br>Specificity 71.3%[18]<br>Odds ratio 3.00[18] |
| Polygonal lines coalescing to form rhomboidal structures | | *Polygonal lines coalescing to form rhomboidal structures* typically surrounding adnexal openings[21] | Sensitivity 16.7%[18]<br>Specificity 91.7%[18]<br>Odds ratio 2[18], 6.18[21] |
| Melanoma of the mucosa — Blue, gray, or white color and a structureless zone | | *Structureless areas contain none of the basic elements such as* dots, globules, circles, or lines. In addition, a lesion with a structureless zone that had blue, gray, or white color was most predictive of melanoma[23] | Sensitivity 100%[23]<br>Specificity 82.2%[23]<br>Odds ratio — |

| | | | |
|---|---|---|---|
| Melanoma of volar surfaces | Parallel ridge pattern | 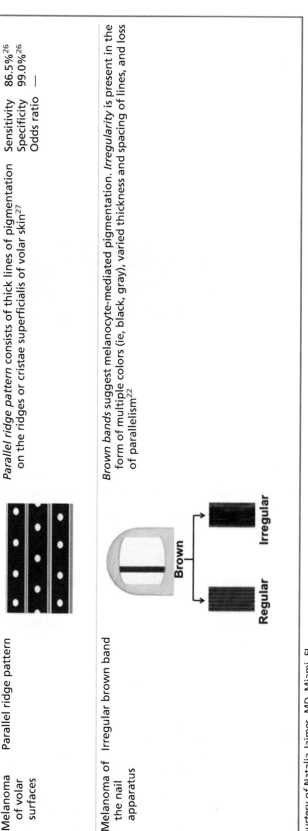 *Parallel ridge pattern* consists of thick lines of pigmentation on the ridges or cristae superficialis of volar skin[27] | Sensitivity 86.5%[26]<br>Specificity 99.0%[26]<br>Odds ratio — |
| Melanoma of the nail apparatus | Irregular brown band | *Brown bands* suggest melanocyte-mediated pigmentation. *Irregularity* is present in the form of multiple colors (ie, black, gray), varied thickness and spacing of lines, and loss of parallelism[22] | |

*Courtesy of Natalia Jaimes, MD, Miami, FL.*

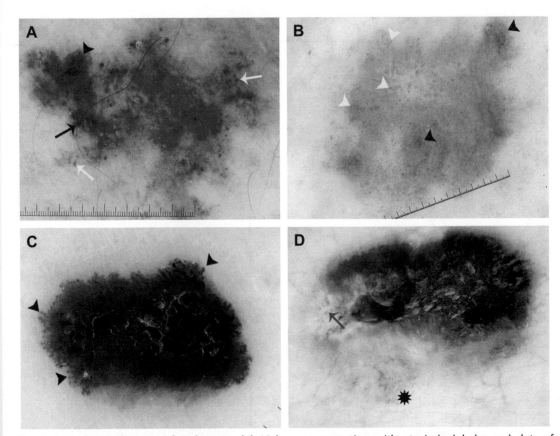

**Fig. 1.** Dermoscopic features of melanoma. (*A*) Melanoma presenting with atypical globules and dots of different sizes and shapes (*yellow arrows*), patches of atypical network (*blue arrowhead*), and a blue-white veil (*blue arrow*). (*B*) Melanoma with diffuse polymorphous vasculature, consisting of serpentine, dotted, and glomerular vessels, can be found throughout the lesion (*yellow arrowheads*). In addition, patches of atypical network (*blue arrowheads*) are seen. (*C*) Superficial spreading melanoma with pseudopods distributed asymmetrically around the lesion (*arrowheads*). (*D*) Melanoma with the regression structure blue-gray peppering (*star*). Shiny white lines are also seen throughout the entire lesion (*red arrows*) along with a central blue-white veil (*red arrowhead*).

## DERMOSCOPIC FEATURES IN ACTINIC KERATOSES, SQUAMOUS CELL CARCINOMA IN SITU/BOWEN DISEASE, INVASIVE SQUAMOUS CELL CARCINOMA, AND KERATOACANTHOMA

Dermoscopic features have been identified that can assist in diagnosing AK, Bowen disease (BD), or in situ squamous cell carcinoma (full-thickness atypia/intraepidermal carcinoma), invasive squamous cell carcinoma (SCC), and keratoacanthoma (KA). Dermoscopically, these lesions exist on a spectrum that the authors have grouped under the category of keratinizing skin cancer (KSC); thus, several features, such as scale, vascular structures, and erythema, are ubiquitous among them. Although more research is needed to determine the sensitivity and specificity of these features, it appears the authors can usually differentiate the full spectrum of KSCs from AKs to IECs to SCCs.

There are several notes that need to be made concerning the data presented in **Tables 4–6**. Many of the lesions examined occur in higher frequency on the head and neck area, thus making generalizability to KSCs on other body parts difficult.[18,35] In addition, several studies look at specific comparisons of the dermoscopic features of AK, for example, to those of SCC, but not all possible diagnoses.[21,36] When a definition was absent from the International Society of Dermoscopy 2016 consensus meeting,[27] the authors cited definitions provided from other sources. Finally, although purported to be significant, some features have yet to be rigorously studied to determine their diagnostic significance. **Tables 4–6** represents the authors' best representation of

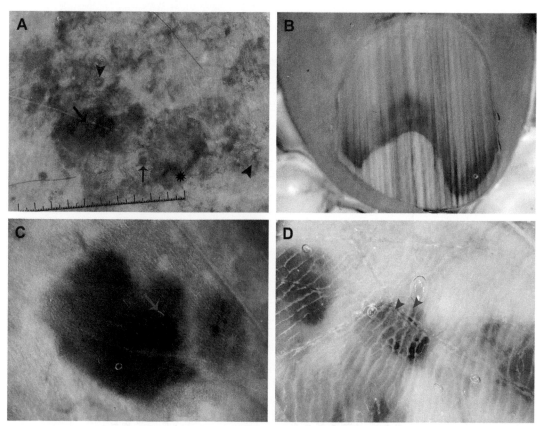

**Fig. 2.** Dermoscopic features of melanoma in special locations. (*A*) LMM on the face with concentric circles, also known as circle within a circle (*blue arrowhead*), gray circles (*blue arrow*), incomplete circles (*black arrowhead*), and angulated lines (*star*). Within the melanoma, there is a seborrheic keratosis (*black arrow*) with comedo-like openings. (*B*) Melanoma of the nail matrix with brown lines that vary in thickness and have a disruption in parallelism. The patient has distal onycholysis. (*C*) Melanoma of the vulva with a linear pattern with features resembling a negative network (*asterisk*). Nevertheless, shiny white structures (*arrow*) and multiple shades of brown with asymmetric distribution of pigment are indicative of melanoma. (*D*) ALM on the volar skin of the heel with pigment on the ridges (*arrowheads*).

available data and, it is hoped, makes clear when little analytical information is known. In addition, examples of dermoscopic features found in KSC are shown in **Fig. 4**.

## DERMOSCOPY ALGORITHMS

Pehamberger and colleagues[37] and Steiner and colleagues[38] first described pattern analysis in dermoscopy as a diagnostic aid to supplement clinical examination of pigmented skin lesions. Pattern analysis is the assessment of the heterogeneity in a pigmented lesion's overall structure, colors, patterns, and margins.[37] Pattern recognition, when used by experts, has been shown to have the best diagnostic performance when compared with other methods[39]; nevertheless, this technique is developed through years of experience. For new users, algorithms are often needed to sift through the diverse array of

presentations of any given type of neoplasm. With the number of new dermoscopy users ever on the increase,[4] along with the inclusion of dermoscopy in national management guidelines,[40–42] algorithms that address skin cancer management as well as diagnosis have become essential.

Although there are multiple algorithms used to teach dermoscopy, the authors rely on the 2-step algorithm.[43] The first step differentiates melanocytic from nonmelanocytic lesions. The second step separates benign from malignant melanocytic lesions.[39] Numerous algorithms have been developed to help new users approach the second step of diagnosing melanoma with high sensitivity and specificity.[44] Some of these algorithms include the ABCD Rule, the 7-point checklist, the Menzies' Method, the CASH algorithm, and the "Chaos and Clues" algorithm.[7,45–48] The latter emphasizes the importance of a disorganized distribution of dermoscopic structures in

**Table 3**
Classic features of basal cell carcinomas

| Dermoscopic Structures | Schematic Illustration | Definition | Diagnostic Value | |
|---|---|---|---|---|
| Spoke-wheel areas, concentric structures (clod within a clod), and leaflike areas | | *Spoke-wheel areas* are brown to blue/gray well-circumscribed radial projections that originate from a central darker hub.[27] If individual radial projections are not visible, then this structure will appear as a concentric globular structure where the center of the globule will appear darker<br>*Leaflike areas*, considered to be a similar structure to spoke-wheel areas, are brown to blue/gray bulbous projections that coalesce into a darker off-center base. This structure often resembles the shape of a leaf[27] | Sensitivity | 10%–17%[31] |
| | | | Specificity | 100%[31] |
| | | | Odds ratio | — |
| Multiple blue-gray nonaggregated dots and globules and large blue-gray ovoid nests | | *Blue-gray dots* in BCC have a buck-shot distribution pattern.<br>*Blue-gray globules* are well-circumscribed oval structures that are distributed in a nonaggregated pattern[66]<br>*Blue-gray ovoid nests* are larger than globules and encompass at least 10% of the surface area of the lesion. They are well-circumscribed structures with a confluent to nearly confluent color[27,66] | Sensitivity | 27%[31]; 55%[31] |
| | | | Specificity | 97%[31]; 99%[31] |
| | | | Odds ratio | — |

| Feature | Image | Description | Statistics | |
|---|---|---|---|---|
| Arborizing (branched) vessels | | Large-caliber vessels that branch into thinner vessels. They are sharply in focus and bright red in color[27] | Sensitivity<br>Specificity<br>Odds ratio | 20%[36], 52%[31], 72%[67]<br>92%–100%[31,36,67]<br>6.7[36] |
| Ulceration | | A structureless area with a red-orange color that may have a serous crust.[66] Smaller ulcers grouped together are known as multiple small erosions | Sensitivity<br>Specificity<br>Odds ratio | 27%[31]<br>97%[31]<br>— |
| Short fine vessels | | Short (<1 mm), thin, linear vessels with little to no branching points.[66] These vessels are more frequently found in superficial BCCs when compared with nodular BCCs[68,69] | | |
| Shiny white blotches and strands | | Shiny white blotches and strands appear shiny white under polarized light, a feature common across all shiny white structures. Unique to BCC are shiny white structures in the shape of blotches and strands[27,33] | | |

*Data from* Menzies SW, Westerhoff K, Rabinovitz H, et al. Surface microscopy of pigmented basal cell carcinoma. Arch Dermatol 2000;136(8):1012–6; and Courtesy of Natalia Jaimes, MD, Miami, FL.

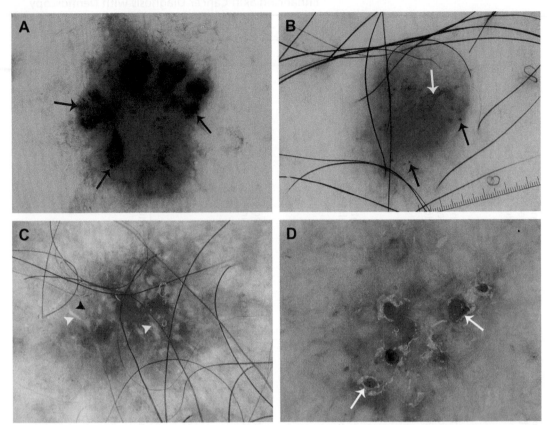

**Fig. 3.** Dermoscopic features of BCC. (*A*) Pigmented BCC with leaflike structures (*black arrow*) and blue-gray ovoid nests, globules, and dots (*blue arrows*). (*B*) Nodular BCC with an arborizing vessel (*yellow arrow*) and blue-gray dots and globules (*blue arrows*). (*C*) Nonpigmented superficial BCC with shiny white blotches and strands (*yellow arrowheads*) and short fine vessels (*blue arrowhead*). (*D*) Superficial BCC with multiple erosions/ulcerations (*arrows*) over an erythematous background with polymorphous vessels.

| Table 4 Actinic keratoses | | | |
|---|---|---|---|
| **Pigmented Tumors** | | | |
| Dermoscopic Structures | Schematic Illustration | Definition/Significance | Diagnostic Value |
| Strawberry pattern | | *Strawberry pattern* is a red pseudonetwork (background erythema and fine wavy vessels) punctuated by adnexal openings accentuated by a white halo.[27] A study comparing actinic keratoses to lentigo maligna demonstrated the preservation of follicle integrity is 12.45 times more likely of being pigmented actinic keratosis[21] | Sensitivity 95.6%[70] Specificity 95.0%[70] Odds ratio 3.6; 13.52[21] |
| Surface scale | | *Surface* scale consists of homogenous opaque adherently keratotic structures with yellowish to brown or white coloration.[70,71] It is a common feature of actinic keratosis and SCC[35] | Sensitivity 93.7%[70]; 37.7%[18] Specificity 35%[70]; 94.2%[18] Odds ratio 7.67[21]; 3.4 (relative risk, RR)[18] |

*Courtesy of* Natalia Jaimes, MD, Miami, FL.

**Table 5**
**Intraepidermal carcinoma and squamous cell carcinoma**

| Dermoscopic Structures | Schematic Illustration | Definition/Significance | Diagnostic Value |
|---|---|---|---|
| **Pigmented tumors** | | | |
| Globules/dots or round circles | | *Globules/dots or round circles* are brown to gray structures that, when arranged in a linear fashion, were frequently found in pigmented intraepidermal carcinoma[72] | |
| **Nonpigmented tumors** | | | |
| Ulceration | | *Ulceration* includes large structureless area with dark red to brown coloration with a serous crust. Classically attributed and identified in SCC, but no studies have determined sensitivity or specificity.[35,71] "Blood spots" have been identified as independent positive predictors of KAs and SCCs, yet an association with ulceration remains unevaluated[73] | |
| Rosettes | | *Rosettes* consist of 4 bright white clods or dots arranged in a 2-by-2 pattern, also called a 4-leaf-clover pattern. This structure can only be seen with polarized light and corresponds to keratin-filled adnexal openings that are most commonly seen in actinically damaged skin, actinic keratosis, and SCC[27,33,74] | |
| Glomerular vessels | | *Glomerular or coiled vessels* are often seen in SCC.[27,75] The presence of clustering of glomerular, dotted, and irregular vessels is highly associated with intraepidermal carcinoma[36] | Sensitivity 60%[36]; 27%[67] <br> Specificity 94%[36]; 100%[67] <br> Odds ratio 21.9[36] |
| Polymorphous vasculature | | *Polymorphous vasculature* is an array of multiple (looped, dotted, and/or serpentine) vessels distributed irregularly throughout the lesion.[27] Classically, this pattern is associated with SCC, but no studies have evaluated sensitivity/specificity of the polymorphous pattern.[35,76] Increasing vascularity, higher vessels' caliber, and visible bleeding were significantly associated with poorly differentiated SCC[77] | |

*Courtesy of* Natalia Jaimes, MD, Miami, FL.

malignant lesions.[7] Although on rare occasions skin cancers lack disorganization, they can usually be identified based on the presence of a starburst-like pattern, negative network, shiny white structures, and polymorphous vessels. Although the aforementioned algorithms have served us well, there is still a need for simpler triage algorithms that can aid beginners in effectively screening for malignancies. Multiple attempts have been made to create a simplified triage algorithm.[7,45–48] The triage amalgamated dermoscopy algorithm (TADA) is a new algorithm that attempts to provide a comprehensive approach to dermoscopy-guided management of pigmented and nonpigmented skin cancers through a combination of previously validated criteria and features (**Fig. 5**).[19,32,49–54] A novel aspect of TADA is that it first asks users to determine if a lesion is an

**Table 6**
**Keratoacanthoma and/or well-differentiated squamous cell carcinoma**

| Dermoscopic Structures | Schematic Illustration | Definition/Significance | Diagnostic Value | |
|---|---|---|---|---|
| White circles | | *White circles* are bright white circles surrounding a dilated infundibulum filled with a yellow/orange keratin plug.[73] This structure is associated with well-differentiated SCC and often seen in KAs[73] | Sensitivity | 31.9%[18] |
| | | | Specificity | 94.2%[18] |
| | | | Odds ratio | 3.0 (RR)[18] |
| Looped vessels | | *Looped vessels* are vascular loops that, depending on the dermoscopy user's angle of view, can appear twisted.[27] Looped vessels have been observed in higher frequencies in nodular SCC and KAs[35,73,78] | | |

*Courtesy of* Natalia Jaimes, MD, Miami, FL.

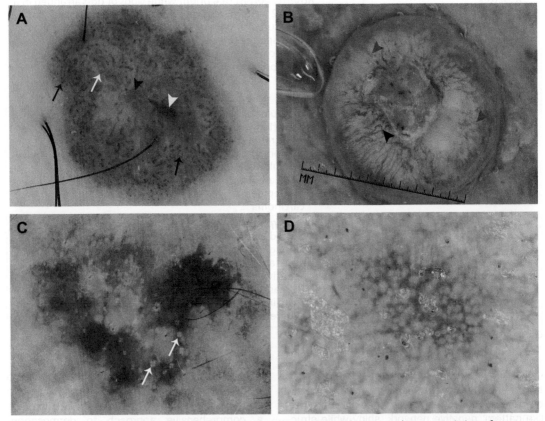

**Fig. 4.** Dermoscopic features of KSCs. (*A*) SCC showing diffuse polymorphous vasculature consisting of numerous serpentine (*black arrow*), dotted (*blue arrow*), and looped vessels (*yellow arrow*). A triangular ulceration (*yellow arrowhead*) with associated scale (*blue arrowhead*) is also seen. (*B*) KA presenting with a central keratin plug and a peripheral rim of irregular looped (*red arrowheads*) and serpentine vessels (*black arrowhead*). (*C*) Pigmented SCC with numerous rosettes (*arrows*). (*D*) Actinic keratosis with a strawberry pattern consisting of a structureless red area interrupted by the follicular openings.

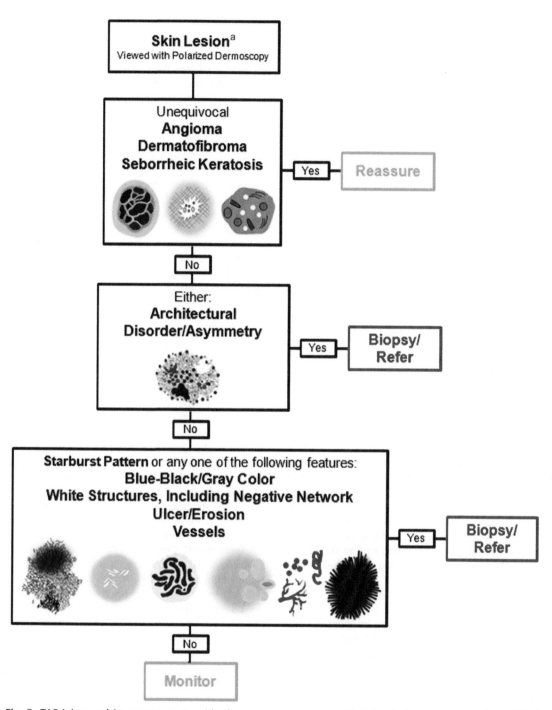

**Fig. 5.** TADA is a multistep process to guide dermoscopic management of skin lesions. First, unequivocal angiomas, dermatofibromas, and seborrheic keratoses are identified and excluded from further evaluation. Next, the lesion is evaluated for the presence of architectural disorder or order. If architectural disorder is present, the lesion should be biopsied or referred for further management. On rare occasion, a malignancy can present in an organized fashion; thus, all organized lesions are then evaluated for blue-black or gray color, white structures, negative network, ulcer/erosion, starburst pattern, and/or vessels. The presence of any one of these features would raise concern for malignancy. [a] Lesions of the volar surfaces, nails, mucosal surfaces, and face should not be evaluated with this algorithm. (*Courtesy of* Natalia Jaimes, MD, Miami, FL; Zachary J. Wolner, BA, Oriol Yelamos, MD, Konstantinos Liopyris, MD, Tova Rogers, MFA, Michael A. Marchetti, MD, Ashfaq A. Marghoob, MD, New York, NY.)

unequivocal example of a dermatofibroma, angioma, and seborrheic keratosis. If the user is confident that the lesions are one of these three, it is excluded from further evaluation with the algorithm. The TADA algorithm is not meant to evaluate lesions on the palms, soles, or nails.

The second step of TADA asks users to evaluate architectural disorder. A study led by the International Dermoscopy Society found architectural disorder, with an odds ratio of 6.6, the most powerful discriminator of melanoma.[44] Furthermore, the subjective interpretation of architectural disorder had the highest interobserver agreement among participants (intraclass correlation coefficient [ICC] of 0.43, where an ICC of 0 is an agreement by chance and an ICC of 1 is perfect agreement).[44] The additional criteria included in TADA (starburst pattern, blue-black or gray color, shiny white structures, negative network, ulcer/erosion, and/or vessels) are needed to identify organized-appearing malignancies, such as spitzoid, nodular, and amelanotic melanoma. The presence of any one feature indicates the need for a biopsy or specialist referral.

In a pilot study, novice dermoscopy users were able to achieve a 93.3% sensitivity and 74.1% specificity using TADA for the identification of malignant study lesions (melanoma, BCC, SCC) after 1 day of dermoscopy training.[55] The high sensitivity seen with TADA was at the expense of specificity; however, the values seen in this study were still equivalent or better than those reported for existing triage algorithms.[39] Thus, with a minor increase in biopsies and referrals for unequivocal lesions, fewer malignant lesions will be missed. TADA has the remarkable potential for enhancing skin cancer screening and detection among individuals with limited dermoscopy training and experience.

## SUMMARY

Dermoscopy has been shown to increase the sensitivity and specificity for diagnosing melanoma. It also enables the diagnosis of melanoma at an earlier stage. In addition, several studies have established dermoscopy as a diagnostic aid for BCC and more recently in clinically determining its histopathological subtype. AK, BD, IEC, SCC, and KA share common dermoscopic features, although multiple specific features have been described allowing accurate diagnosis of specific tumors. Diagnostic algorithms are often used to aid in the dermoscopic evaluation and diagnosis of skin lesions. The advent of triage algorithms can assist beginners with determining if a lesion requires a biopsy or specialist referral without having to arrive at a specific diagnosis. TADA is one

such algorithm that includes a limited set of dermoscopic features and can thus be easily learned and implemented by new users. The features included in TADA were selected for their abilities to discriminate a wider range of common pigmented and nonpigmented skin cancers.

## REFERENCES

1. Carli P, De Giorgi V, Crocetti E, et al. Improvement of malignant/benign ratio in excised melanocytic lesions in the 'dermoscopy era': a retrospective study 1997-2001. Br J Dermatol 2004;150(4):687–92.
2. Vestergaard M, Macaskill P, Holt P, et al. Dermoscopy compared with naked eye examination for the diagnosis of primary melanoma: a meta-analysis of studies performed in a clinical setting. Br J Dermatol 2008;159(3):669–76.
3. Salerni G, Teran T, Puig S, et al. Meta-analysis of digital dermoscopy follow-up of melanocytic skin lesions: a study on behalf of the International Dermoscopy Society. J Eur Acad Dermatol Venereol 2013;27(7):805–14.
4. Terushkin V, Oliveria SA, Marghoob AA, et al. Use of and beliefs about total body photography and dermatoscopy among US dermatology training programs: an update. J Am Acad Dermatol 2010;62(5):794–803.
5. Nehal KS, Oliveria SA, Marghoob AA, et al. Use of and beliefs about baseline photography in the management of patients with pigmented lesions: a survey of dermatology residency programmes in the United States. Melanoma Res 2002;12(2):161–7.
6. Argenziano G, Puig S, Zalaudek I, et al. Dermoscopy improves accuracy of primary care physicians to triage lesions suggestive of skin cancer. J Clin Oncol 2006;24(12):1877–82.
7. Rosendahl C, Cameron A, McColl I, et al. Dermatoscopy in routine practice - 'chaos and clues'. Aust Fam Physician 2012;41(7):482–7.
8. Haspeslagh M, Vossaert K, Lanssens S, et al. Comparison of ex vivo and in vivo dermoscopy in dermatopathologic evaluation of skin tumors. JAMA Dermatol 2016;152(3):312–7.
9. Bafounta M, Beauchet A, Aegerter P, et al. Is dermoscopy (epiluminescence microscopy) useful for the diagnosis of melanoma? Results of a meta-analysis using techniques adapted to the evaluation of diagnostic tests. Arch Dermatol 2001; 137(10):1343–50.
10. Kittler H, Pehamberger H, Wolff K, et al. Diagnostic accuracy of dermoscopy. Lancet Oncol 2002;3(3): 159–65.
11. Terushkin V, Warycha M, Levy M, et al. Analysis of the benign to malignant ratio of lesions biopsied by a general dermatologist before and after the adoption of dermoscopy. Arch Dermatol 2010; 146(3):343–4.

12. Binder M, Puespoeck-Schwarz M, Steiner A, et al. Epiluminescence microscopy of small pigmented skin lesions: short-term formal training improves the diagnostic performance of dermatologists. J Am Acad Dermatol 1997;36(2):197–202.

13. Chen L, Liebman T, Soriano R, et al. One-year follow-up of dermoscopy education on the ability of medical students to detect skin cancer. Dermatology 2013;226(3):267–73.

14. Carli P, de Giorgi V, Chiarugi A, et al. Addition of dermoscopy to conventional naked-eye examination in melanoma screening: a randomized study. J Am Acad Dermatol 2004;50(5):683–9.

15. Argenziano G, Cerroni L, Zalaudek I, et al. Accuracy in melanoma detection: a 10-year multicenter survey. J Am Acad Dermatol 2012;67(1):54–9.

16. Haenssle H, Hoffmann S, Holzkamp R, et al. Melanoma thickness: the role of patients' characteristics, risk indicators and patterns of diagnosis. J Eur Acad Dermatol Venereol 2015;29(1):102–8.

17. Yadav S, Vossaert K, Kopf A, et al. Histopathologic correlates of structures seen on dermoscopy (epiluminescence microscopy). Am J Dermatopathol 1993;15(4):297–305.

18. Tschandl P, Rosendahl C, Kittler H. Dermatoscopy of flat pigmented facial lesions. J Eur Acad Dermatol Venereol 2015;29(1):120–7.

19. Marghoob AA, Braun R, Malvehy J, editors. Atlas of dermoscopy. 2nd edition. London: Informa Healthcare; 2012.

20. Schiffner R, Schiffner-Rohe J, Vogt T, et al. Improvement of early recognition of lentigo maligna using dermatoscopy. J Am Acad Dermatol 2000; 42(1 Pt 1):25–32.

21. Lallas A, Tschandl P, Kyrgidis A, et al. Dermoscopic clues to differentiate facial lentigo maligna from pigmented actinic keratosis. Br J Dermatol 2016;174(5): 1079–85.

22. Braun RP, Baran R, Le Gal FA, et al. Diagnosis and management of nail pigmentations. J Am Acad Dermatol 2007;56(5):835–47.

23. Blum A, Simionescu O, Argenziano G, et al. Dermoscopy of pigmented lesions of the mucosa and the mucocutaneous junction: results of a multicenter study by the International Dermoscopy Society (IDS). Arch Dermatol 2011;147(10):1181–7.

24. Lin J, Koga H, Takata M, et al. Dermoscopy of pigmented lesions on mucocutaneous junction and mucous membrane. Br J Dermatol 2009;161(6):1255–61.

25. Saida T, Koga H, Goto Y, et al. Characteristic distribution of melanin columns in the cornified layer of acquired acral nevus: an important clue for histopathologic differentiation from early acral melanoma. Am J Dermatopathol 2011;33(5):468–73.

26. Saida T, Miyazaki A, Oguchi S, et al. Significance of dermoscopic patterns in detecting malignant melanoma on acral volar skin: results of a multicenter study in Japan. Arch Dermatol 2004;140(10): 1233–8.

27. Kittler H, Marghoob AA, Argenziano G, et al. Standardization of terminology in dermoscopy/dermatoscopy: results of the third consensus conference of the International Society of Dermoscopy. J Am Acad Dermatol 2016;74(6):1093–106.

28. Rosendahl C, Tschandl P, Cameron A, et al. Diagnostic accuracy of dermatoscopy for melanocytic and nonmelanocytic pigmented lesions. J Am Acad Dermatol 2011;64(6):1068–73.

29. Ahnlide I, Zalaudek I, Nilsson F, et al. Preoperative prediction of histopathological outcome in basal cell carcinoma: flat surface and multiple small erosions predict superficial basal cell carcinoma in lighter skin types. Br J Dermatol 2016;175(4): 751–61.

30. Lallas A, Argenziano G, Kyrgidis A, et al. Dermoscopy uncovers clinically undetectable pigmentation in basal cell carcinoma. Br J Dermatol 2014; 170(1):192–5.

31. Menzies SW, Westerhoff K, Rabinovitz H, et al. Surface microscopy of pigmented basal cell carcinoma. Arch Dermatol 2000;136(8):1012–6.

32. Altamura D, Menzies SW, Argenziano G, et al. Dermatoscopy of basal cell carcinoma: morphologic variability of global and local features and accuracy of diagnosis. J Am Acad Dermatol 2010; 62(1):67–75.

33. Liebman TN, Rabinovitz HS, Dusza SW, et al. White shiny structures: dermoscopic features revealed under polarized light. J Eur Acad Dermatol Venereol 2012;26(12):1493–7.

34. Lallas A, Tzellos T, Kyrgidis A, et al. Accuracy of dermoscopic criteria for discriminating superficial from other subtypes of basal cell carcinoma. J Am Acad Dermatol 2014;70(2):303–11.

35. Zalaudek I, Giacomel J, Schmid K, et al. Dermatoscopy of facial actinic keratosis, intraepidermal carcinoma, and invasive squamous cell carcinoma: a progression model. J Am Acad Dermatol 2012; 66(4):589–97.

36. Pan Y, Chamberlain AJ, Bailey M, et al. Dermatoscopy aids in the diagnosis of the solitary red scaly patch or plaque-features distinguishing superficial basal cell carcinoma, intraepidermal carcinoma, and psoriasis. J Am Acad Dermatol 2008;59(2): 268–74.

37. Pehamberger H, Steiner A, Wolff K. In vivo epiluminescence microscopy of pigmented skin lesions. I. Pattern analysis of pigmented skin lesions. J Am Acad Dermatol 1987;17(4):571–83.

38. Steiner A, Pehamberger H, Wolff K. In vivo epiluminescence microscopy of pigmented skin lesions. II. Diagnosis of small pigmented skin lesions and early detection of malignant melanoma. J Am Acad Dermatol 1987;17(4):584–91.

39. Argenziano G, Soyer HP, Chimenti S, et al. Dermoscopy of pigmented skin lesions: results of a consensus meeting via the Internet. J Am Acad Dermatol 2003;48(5):679–93.

40. Dummer R, Hauschild A, Lindenblatt N, et al. Cutaneous melanoma: ESMO Clinical Practice Guidelines for diagnosis, treatment and follow-up. Ann Oncol 2015;26(suppl 5):v126–32.

41. Marsden J, Newton-Bishop J, Burrows L, et al. Revised U.K. guidelines for the management of cutaneous melanoma 2010. Br J Dermatol 2010; 163(2):238–56.

42. Garbe C, Peris K, Hauschild A, et al. Diagnosis and treatment of melanoma. European consensus-based interdisciplinary guideline - Update 2016. Eur J Cancer 2016;63:201–17.

43. Kittler H. The 2-Step method and the recognition process in dermoscopy. JAMA Dermatol 2015; 151(9):1037–8.

44. Carrera C, Marchetti MA, Dusza SW, et al. Validity and reliability of dermoscopic criteria used to differentiate nevi from melanoma: a web-based International Dermoscopy Society Study. JAMA Dermatol 2016;152(7):798–806.

45. Argenziano G, Fabbrocini G, Carli P, et al. Epiluminescence microscopy for the diagnosis of doubtful melanocytic skin lesions. Comparison of the ABCD rule of dermatoscopy and a new 7-point checklist based on pattern analysis. Arch Dermatol 1998; 134(12):1563–70.

46. Soyer HP, Argenziano G, Zalaudek I, et al. Three-point checklist of dermoscopy. A new screening method for early detection of melanoma. Dermatology 2004;208(1):27–31.

47. Henning JS, Dusza SW, Wang SQ, et al. The CASH (color, architecture, symmetry, and homogeneity) algorithm for dermoscopy. J Am Acad Dermatol 2007; 56(1):45–52.

48. Stolz W, Riemann A, Cognetta A, et al. ABCD rule of dermoscopy: a new practical method for early recognition of malignant melanoma. Eur J Dermatol 1994;(4):521–7.

49. Marghoob AA, Usatine RP, Jaimes N. Dermoscopy for the family physician. Am Fam Physician 2013; 88(7):441–50.

50. Lallas A, Moscarella E, Longo C, et al. Likelihood of finding melanoma when removing a Spitzoid-looking lesion in patients aged 12 years or older. J Am Acad Dermatol 2015;72(1):47–53.

51. Argenziano G, Longo C, Cameron A, et al. Blue-black rule: a simple dermoscopic clue to recognize pigmented nodular melanoma. Br J Dermatol 2011; 165(6):1251–5.

52. Zalaudek I, Kittler H, Hofmann-Wellenhof R, et al. "White" network in Spitz nevi and early melanomas lacking significant pigmentation. J Am Acad Dermatol 2013;69(1):56–60.

53. Balagula Y, Braun R, Rabinovitz H, et al. The significance of crystalline/chrysalis structures in the diagnosis of melanocytic and nonmelanocytic lesions. J Am Acad Dermatol 2012;67(2):194.e1-8.

54. Pizzichetta MA, Talamini R, Marghoob AA, et al. Negative pigment network: an additional dermoscopic feature for the diagnosis of melanoma. J Am Acad Dermatol 2013;68(4):552–9.

55. Rogers T, Marino ML, Dusza SW, et al. A clinical aid for detecting skin cancer: the triage amalgamated dermoscopic algorithm (TADA). J Am Board Fam Med 2016;29(6):694–701.

56. Argenziano G, Fabbrocini G, Carli P, et al. Epiluminescence microscopy: criteria of cutaneous melanoma progression. J Am Acad Dermatol 1997; 37(1):68–74.

57. Menzies SW, Kreusch J, Byth K, et al. Dermoscopic evaluation of amelanotic and hypomelanotic melanoma. Arch Dermatol 2008;144(9): 1120–7.

58. Salopek TG, Kopf AW, Stefanato CM, et al. Differentiation of atypical moles (dysplastic nevi) from early melanomas by dermoscopy. Dermatol Clin 2001; 19(2):337–45.

59. Soyer HP, Smolle J, Leitinger G, et al. Diagnostic reliability of dermoscopic criteria for detecting malignant melanoma. Dermatology 1995;190(1): 25–30.

60. Annessi G, Bon R, Sampogna F, et al. Sensitivity, specificity, and diagnostic accuracy of three dermoscopic algorithmic methods in the diagnosis of doubtful melanocytic lesions: the importance of light brown structureless areas in differentiating atypical melanocytic nevi from thin melanomas. J Am Acad Dermatol 2007;56(5):759–67.

61. Haenssle HA, Korpas B, Hansen-Hagge C, et al. Seven-point checklist for dermatoscopy: performance during 10 years of prospective surveillance of patients at increased melanoma risk. J Am Acad Dermatol 2010;62(5):785–93.

62. Menzies SW, Ingvar C, McCarthy WH. A sensitivity and specificity analysis of the surface microscopy features of invasive melanoma. Melanoma Res 1996;6(1):55–62.

63. Kenet RO, Kang S, Kenet BJ, et al. Clinical diagnosis of pigmented lesions using digital epiluminescence microscopy. Grading protocol and atlas. Arch Dermatol 1993;129(2):157–74.

64. Bassoli S, Ferrari C, Borsari S, et al. Negative pigment network identifies a peculiar melanoma subtype and represents a clue to melanoma diagnosis: a dermoscopic study of 401 melanomas. Acta Derm Venereol 2013;93(6):650–5.

65. Alon S, Katrin K, Harold SR. Histopathologic tissue correlations of dermoscopic structures. An atlas of dermoscopy. 2nd edition. New York: CRC Press; 2012. p. 10–32.

66. Lallas A, Apalla Z, Argenziano G, et al. The dermatoscopic universe of basal cell carcinoma. Dermatol Pract Concept 2014;4(3):11–24.

67. Sakakibara A, Kamijima M, Shibata S, et al. Dermoscopic evaluation of vascular structures of various skin tumors in Japanese patients. J Dermatol 2010; 37(4):316–22.

68. Micantonio T, Gulia A, Altobelli E, et al. Vascular patterns in basal cell carcinoma. J Eur Acad Dermatol Venereol 2011;25(3):358–61.

69. Giacomel J, Zalaudek I. Dermoscopy of superficial basal cell carcinoma. Dermatol Surg 2005;31(12): 1710–3.

70. Huerta-Brogeras M, Olmos O, Borbujo J, et al. Validation of dermoscopy as a real-time noninvasive diagnostic imaging technique for actinic keratosis. Arch Dermatol 2012;148(10):1159–64.

71. Fargnoli MC, Kostaki D, Piccioni A, et al. Dermoscopy in the diagnosis and management of nonmelanoma skin cancers. Eur J Dermatol 2012; 22(4):456–63.

72. Cameron A, Rosendahl C, Tschandl P, et al. Dermatoscopy of pigmented Bowen's disease. J Am Acad Dermatol 2010;62(4):597–604.

73. Rosendahl C, Cameron A, Argenziano G, et al. Dermoscopy of squamous cell carcinoma and keratoacanthoma. Arch Dermatol 2012;148(12): 1386–92.

74. Cuellar F, Vilalta A, Puig S, et al. New dermoscopic pattern in actinic keratosis and related conditions. Arch Dermatol 2009;145(6):732.

75. Argenziano G, Zalaudek I, Corona R, et al. Vascular structures in skin tumors: a dermoscopy study. Arch Dermatol 2004;140(12):1485–9.

76. Zalaudek II. How to diagnose nonpigmented skin tumors: a review of vascular structures seen with dermoscopy: part II. Nonmelanocytic skin tumors. J Am Acad Dermatol 2010;63(3):377–86 [quiz: 387–8].

77. Lallas A, Pyne J, Kyrgidis A, et al. The clinical and dermoscopic features of invasive cutaneous squamous cell carcinoma depend on the histopathological grade of differentiation. Br J Dermatol 2015; 172(5):1308–15.

78. Lin MJ, Pan Y, Jalilian C, et al. Dermoscopic characteristics of nodular squamous cell carcinoma and keratoacanthoma. Dermatol Pract Concept 2014; 4(2):9–15.

# Mole Mapping for Management of Pigmented Skin Lesions

Juliana Berk-Krauss, BA[a,b], David Polsky, MD, PhD[b],
Jennifer A. Stein, MD, PhD[b,*]

## KEYWORDS

- Melanoma screening • Dermoscopy • Mole mapping • Total-body photography
- Sequential digital dermoscopy imaging • Digital follow-up

## KEY POINTS

- Detecting melanoma, particularly in patients with numerous or atypical nevi, can be challenging for even the most skilled dermatologists.
- Mole mapping involves using noninvasive imaging technology to enhance monitoring of new or changing melanocytic lesions.
- Total-body photography and sequential digital dermoscopy imaging, together known as digital follow-up, are 2 prominent forms of noninvasive imaging technology used in mole mapping.
- Noninvasive imaging technologies have been found to improve diagnostic accuracy, detect earlier-stage melanomas, and reduce costs.
- Total-body photography and sequential digital dermoscopy imaging, in combination with direct-to-consumer applications and teledermatology, are already revolutionizing the ways in which physicians and patients participate in melanoma surveillance and will likely continue to enhance early detection efforts.

## INTRODUCTION

The incidence of cutaneous malignant melanoma is increasing at a rate faster than any of the other 5 most common cancers in the United States.[1] Approximately 76,380 cases of melanoma and 10,130 deaths are expected in 2016.[2] Because of the inverse relationship between primary tumor thickness and survival time, effective early detection of melanoma remains one of the most crucial strategies in improving patient prognosis.[3] Dermatologists have traditionally screened for melanoma using a combination of clinical evaluation and dermoscopy (epiluminescence microscopy), which is more accurate in diagnosing melanoma than naked-eye examination.[4–6] In patients with numerous or atypical nevi, it can be challenging for detecting new or changing lesions. Mole mapping incorporates photography into melanoma surveillance, making evaluation of multiple and suspicious lesions a more dynamic, objective, and precise process. Total-body photography (TBP)[7,8] and sequential digital dermoscopy imaging (SDDI)[9,10] are 2 prominent forms of noninvasive imaging technology used in mole mapping that have proved helpful in recognizing

Disclosure Statement: The authors have no disclosures to make.
[a] Yale School of Medicine, 333 Cedar Street, New Haven, CT 06510, USA; [b] The Ronald O. Perelman Department of Dermatology, NYU School of Medicine, 240 East 38th Street, 11th Floor, New York, NY 10016, USA
* Corresponding author.
E-mail address: Jennifer.Stein@nyumc.org

Dermatol Clin 35 (2017) 439–445
http://dx.doi.org/10.1016/j.det.2017.06.004
0733-8635/17/© 2017 Elsevier Inc. All rights reserved.

early-stage melanoma and minimizing benign lesion excisions.

## NONINVASIVE IMAGING TECHNOLOGY CATEGORIES

TBP is a series of approximately 25 images of the entire skin surface that can be used as an adjunct to total-body skin examinations (TBSE), patient self–skin examinations (SSE), and dermoscopy. Photographic documentation serves as a baseline comparison for future TBSEs and allows a physician or patient to detect new lesions and any naked-eye changes in preexisting lesions. Once new or changing lesions have been identified by TBP, dermoscopy and SDDI can be used to further examine a suspicious lesion.

SDDI uses electronic storage of digital dermoscopic images to allow for side-by-side comparison of lesions over time. SDDI enables practitioners to detect changes in structure, color, and size. The electronic storage of digital dermoscopic images can be used for short-term or long-term monitoring. Most centers will use both lengths of follow-up in patients with numerous atypical lesions.[11] Short-term monitoring (approximately 3 months) is useful for detecting subtle changes in a discrete suspicious lesion. This monitoring is typically reserved for flat or only superficially raised lesions that do not satisfy the classic surface microscopic criteria for the diagnosis of melanoma and either

(1) have a recent history of change while exhibiting only minor clinical atypia or (2) are mildly to moderately atypical lesions without a history of change. At follow-up, lesions showing any morphologic change should be excised.[9] Routine long-term monitoring (6–12 months) can be used in patients with numerous lesions thought to be clinically inconspicuous or with other high-risk phenotypes for developing primary melanoma. If asymmetrical enlargement, focal changes in pigmentation and structure, regression features, or change in color (appearance of new colors) are detected during long-term follow-up, excision should be considered. The threshold for excision is commonly determined not only by the morphologic appearance and number of lesions, but also by the patient's skin cancer history, personal preferences, and compliance.[10]

*Digital follow-up* (DFU) refers to the simultaneous implementation of TBP and SDDI[12] (Fig. 1). (For the remainder of this article, mole mapping will be referred to as *DFU*.) Although either TBP or SDDI can be used independently, the combination is superior to a single method alone[13] and when used with SSEs, TBSEs, and dermoscopy, contributes important temporal information to the overall clinical assessment. Lesions with features suggestive of melanoma should undergo biopsy, whereas those with equivocal but not diagnostic features could undergo short-term SDDI.[14]

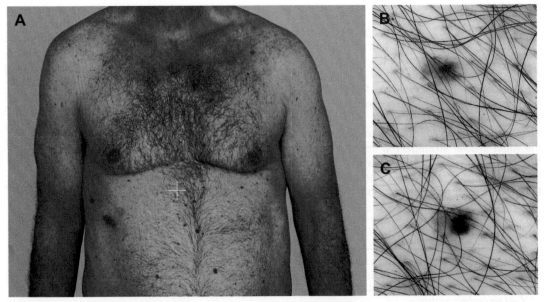

**Fig. 1.** DFU. MoleSafe total body photography (*A*) and sequential digital dermoscopy imaging (*B, C*) of a changing lesion diagnosed as a malignant melanoma in situ (*C*). (*Courtesy of* Juliana Berk-Krauss, BA, David Polsky, MD, PhD, Jennifer Stein MD, PhD, New York, NY.)

## CHALLENGES IN MELANOMA SCREENING

Diagnosis of melanoma is often multifactorial and incorporates patient history, gross and dermoscopic appearance, comparison with neighboring lesions, and identification of change. Although change can be the key and even sole sign of a melanoma,[15] not all new or changing lesions are melanomas.[16] Malignant features are particularly difficult to discern during early stages of melanoma growth, when preventing morbidity and mortality is more likely. One study found that dermoscopists were able to correctly identify small melanomas with only an average diagnostic sensitivity of 39% and a specificity of 82% and recommended small melanomas for biopsy with a sensitivity of 71% and specificity of 49%. Distinguishing between small melanomas and small benign pigmented lesions was difficult for even expert practitioners.[17]

Furthermore, emphasis on detection and subsequent biopsy of changing skin lesions can lead to overdiagnosis, particularly in patients at high risk or with multiple nevi. Benign-to-malignant ratios (the number of biopsies of benign lesions performed to make the diagnosis of one skin cancer) are a helpful measure of diagnostic accuracy. Although there is no clear benchmark, numerous studies have found benign-to-malignant biopsy ratios as low as 3:1 to 30:1 for practitioners using a simple clinical examination to serial photography and dermoscopy.[18,19] The potential for associated harms, such as poor cosmetic results, and increased health care costs with overdiagnosis are real concerns, highlighting the importance of distinguishing truly potentially lethal lesions from those that are benign.[20–22]

## VALUE OF DIGITAL FOLLOW-UP

Noninvasive imaging technology helps dermatologists catch early-stage melanomas while improving diagnostic accuracy.[23,24] As both stand-alone modalities and in combination, TBP and SDDI can confer specific clinical benefits.

TBP is particularly helpful in detecting changes in lesions that often do not follow the classic ABCDE (asymmetry, border irregularity, color variegation, diameter >6 mm, evolving) criteria. Feit and colleagues[25] reported that 74% of melanomas detected in patients with TBP were a result of subtle changes that did not show classical clinical features at the time of detection. On the other hand, TBP can uniquely identify new lesions[26]—in a study of patients with multiple atypical nevi who were undergoing TBP, two-thirds of melanomas detected arose de novo.[24]

SDDI is useful as a second-level screening tool for evaluating lesions with borderline features.[27] Using SDDI in these scenarios, physicians have the option of resorting to short-term follow-up, when they might have otherwise biopsied a lesion. SDDI also allows sensitive detection of the most relevant and often subtle microscopic changes associated with melanoma, such as the development of new focal or eccentric new structures, atypical vessels, regression features, or asymmetric enlargement[14] (Fig. 2).

Multiple studies found the advantage of SDDI when used for patients who have risk factors predisposing them to melanoma.[13] Commonly used inclusion criteria are the presence of atypical mole syndrome, numerous nevi, atypical nevi, genetic mutations (ie, CDKN2A), and personal or familial history of melanoma. The increase in risk carried with each one of these factors can range from 1.5- to 10-fold.[28] When low-risk patients were included in a cohort of SDDI, no melanoma was detected in this subgroup.[29]

In high-risk patients, such as those with atypical mole syndrome, TBP and SDDI used in combination contribute to early detection of melanomas with a low rate of excisions.[11,30] Numerous meta-analyses strongly suggest that the use of DFU and dermoscopy to identify and evaluate new or changing skin lesions permits physicians to diagnose melanomas at curable stages with low benign/malignant biopsy ratios.[5,13] Additionally, TBP images, often provided for patients to take home, have been found to augment patient SSEs. Use of TBP images during SSEs increases frequency of SSEs, improves patient confidence in performing them, and enhances their detection sensitivity.[31] The combination of these effects ultimately decreases cancer worry.[32]

DFU not only serves as an opportunity to provide patients with a high quality of care but also has the potential to relieve the health care system of some financial burden. In minimizing excision rates, imaging modalities are cost saving in patients with numerous or atypical nevi. A 1-year retrospective observational study in Belgium found that SDDI resulted in a 35% reduction in the cost per melanoma excised compared with dermoscopy alone.[33] An Australian study that used TBP in high-risk patients, found that prophylactically excising all 5838 clinically atypical nevi in the study would have cost more than 1 million Australian dollars in 1987. The actual cost was AU$5583 (AU$100/set of photos).[24]

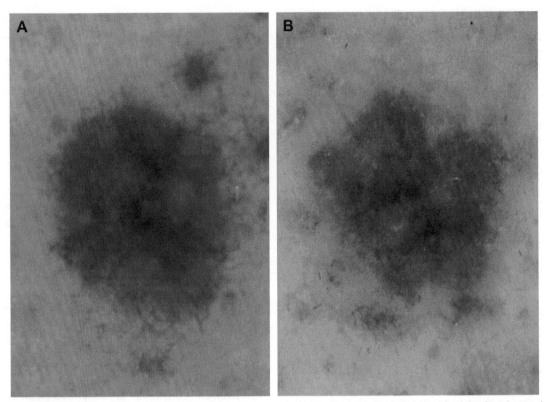

**Fig. 2.** Short-term monitoring with sequential digital dermoscopy imaging. Baseline image (*A*) of a changed lesion diagnosed as a 0.3-mm melanoma (*B*). (*Courtesy of* Juliana Berk-Krauss, BA, David Polsky, MD, PhD, Jennifer Stein MD, PhD, New York, NY.)

## DIGITAL FOLLOW-UP EXPANSION

Since the advent of TBP in the late 1980s, noninvasive imaging technology has steadily grown.[7] In 2000, 62% of dermatologists in academic institutions reported using TBP. In 2010, this proportion increased to 71%.[34] That same year, a study surveying 49 US dermatology departments found two-thirds use TBP as a screening method. Of those who used TBP, one-third used digital TBP alone, one-third used digital with printed images of TBP, and the last third used printed TBP images alone.[35] In 2013, 49.3% of US dermatologists reported using SDDI.[36] In Europe and Australia, the use of dermoscopy and SDDI is thought to be common practice among an most dermatologists.[14]

The types of DFU systems range from simple to highly advanced photography. Numerous medical imaging companies are entering this expanding market with DFU products. Some examples include MoleSafe, DermSpectra, Foto-Finder, and Canfield, which all use TBP systems that digitally link to dermoscopic images of lesions of interest. However, they each provide variations of photography sites (imaging centers vs physician office), photographers (professional vs medical personnel), hardware, and software.

MoleSafe is unique in that the final report, which comprises the complete skin record with digital images and clinical information, is reviewed by an expert physician dermoscopist before being sent to the referring physician and patient, thus effectively incorporating DFU with teledermatology.[37] Canfield provides 3-dimensional TBP, which uses a fixed array of cameras and specialized software to process and assemble a 3-dimensionsl digital model of the patient showing the entire skin surface linked to 2-dimensional dermoscopy.[38]

## CURRENT CHALLENGES AND FUTURE DIRECTIONS OF DIGITAL FOLLOW-UP

Despite the impressive advances in this field, it seems that imaging modalities are concentrated largely in academic centers treating high-risk patients.[36] More work needs to be done to improve usability and access to DFU. Limitations to using these new technologies include logistical constraints—additional time required and secure software to organize and store images—lack of knowledge regarding the utility of the technique, lack of training, and cost.[34,39]

DFU is perceived by many dermatologists to make the clinical examination slower.[34] In one study, the median time needed for TBSE without dermoscopy was half as long as with simple dermoscopy and was in direct proportion to the patient's total lesion count.[40] Although the technology is becoming increasingly user friendly, imaging training can be tedious and underutilized. Proper use of SDDI reportedly requires 10 to 20 hours of training.[41] A survey of residents in US dermatology training programs found that most thought there was little emphasis on TBP training during residency and that additional training was needed.[34]

For physicians, the equipment and operation requirements for DFU—camera, computer, imaging software, and photographers—can be costly. In a 2009 survey of US dermatologists, half reported that health insurance companies failed to reimburse the cost of TBP.[34] For many patients, TBP is often not covered by insurance, and out of pocket costs can be prohibitive. In some geographic locations, there is simply a paucity of TBP imaging centers, and those that do provide services require hours of preparation, photography time, and follow-up counseling.[14]

These barriers, in concurrence with the advancement of imaging technologies and the development of direct-to-consumer applications and teledermatology, have created a space in which patients can create their own mobile-based TBP and SDDI.[14] A cellphone application developed by Oregon Health & Sciences University called Mole Mapper, allows a patient to use a camera phone to track the clinical appearance of his or her moles over time. The photographs can be shared with their providers and sent to researchers for analysis.[42] Low-cost mobile camera dermatoscope attachments are paving the way for patients to take their own dermoscopic images and participate in teledermoscopy and SDDI with a dermatologist.[41,43] Although these new technologies require further developments in the areas of patient safety and privacy, usability, and quality control, they should continue to be assessed for their role in the early detection of melanoma or follow-up.[44]

## SUMMARY

Identification of melanoma, particularly in patients with numerous or atypical nevi, is a challenge for even the most skilled dermatologists. Augmenting the clinical and dermoscopic examination with TBP and SDDI can improve diagnostic accuracy, detect earlier-stage melanomas, and reduce costs. Although barriers to adoption of these screening techniques exist, it is clear that noninvasive imaging technology is already revolutionizing the ways in which physicians and patients participate in melanoma surveillance and will likely continue to enhance early detection efforts.

## REFERENCES

1. Ryerson AB, Eheman CR, Altekruse SF, et al. Annual report to the Nation on the Status of Cancer, 1975-2012, featuring the increasing incidence of liver cancer. Cancer 2016;122:1332–7.
2. Glazer AM, Winkelmann RR, Farberg AS, et al. Analysis of trends in US melanoma incidence and mortality. JAMA Dermatol 2016. http://dx.doi.org/10.1001/jamadermatol.2016.4512.
3. Breitbart EW, Waldmann A, Nolte S, et al. Systematic skin cancer screening in Northern Germany. J Am Acad Dermatol 2012;66(2):201–11.
4. Soyer HP, Argenziano G, Talamini R, et al. Is dermoscopy useful for the diagnosis of melanoma? Arch Dermatol 2001;137(10):1361–3.
5. Vestergaard ME, Macaskill P, Holt PE, et al. Dermoscopy compared with naked eye examination for the diagnosis of primary melanoma: a meta-analysis of studies performed in a clinical setting. Br J Dermatol 2008;159(3):669–76.
6. Chang Y, Newton-Bishop JA, Bishop DT, et al. A pooled analysis of melanocytic nevus phenotype and the risk of cutaneous melanoma at different latitudes. Int J Cancer 2009;124(2):420–8.
7. Slue W, Kopf AW, Rivers JK. Total-body photographs of dysplastic nevi. Arch Dermatol 1988;124(8):1239–43.
8. Halpern AC. The use of whole body photography in pigmented lesion clinic. Dermatol Surg 2000;26(12):1175–80.
9. Menzies SW, Gutenev A, Avramidis M, et al. Short-term digital surface microscopic monitoring of atypical or changing melanocytic lesions. Arch Dermatol 2001;137(12):1583–9.
10. Kittler H, Guitera P, Riedl E, et al. Identification of clinically featureless incipient melanoma using sequential dermoscopy imaging. Arch Dermatol 2006;142(9):1113–9.
11. Salerni G, Carrera C, Lovatto L, et al. Benefits of total body photography and digital dermatoscopy ("two-step method of digital follow-up") in the early diagnosis of melanoma in patients at high risk for melanoma. J Am Acad Dermatol 2012;67(1):e17–27.
12. Salerni G, Carrera C, Lovatto L, et al. Characterization of 1152 lesions excised over 10 years using total body photography and digital dermoscopy in the

surveillance of patients at high risk for melanoma. J Am Acad Dermatol 2012;67(5):836–45.

13. Salerni G, Teran T, Puig S, et al. Meta-analysis of digital dermoscopy follow-up of melanocytic skin lesions: a study on behalf of the International Dermoscopy Society. J Eur Acad Dermatol Venereol 2013;27(7):805–14.

14. Marino ML, Carrera C, Marchetti MA. Practice gaps in dermatology. Dermatol Clin 2016;34(3):353–62.

15. Abbasi NR, Shaw HM, Rigel DS, et al. Early diagnosis of cutaneous melanoma: revisiting the ABCD criteria. JAMA 2005;292(22):2771–6.

16. Banky JP, Kelly JW, English DR, et al. Incidence of new and changed nevi and melanomas detected using baseline images and dermoscopy in patients at high risk for melanoma. Arch Dermatol 2005; 141(8):998–1006.

17. Friedman RJ, Gutkowicz-Krusin D, Farber MJ. The diagnostic performance of expert dermoscopists vs a computer-vision system on small-diameter melanomas. Arch Dermatol 2008; 144(4):476–82.

18. Soares TF, Laman SD, Yiannias JA, et al. Factors leading to biopsy of 1547 pigmented lesions at Mayo Clinic, Scottsdale, Arizona, in 2005. Int J Dermatol 2009;48(10):1053–6.

19. Koh HK, Norton LA, Geller AC. Evaluation of the American Academy of Dermatology's National skin cancer early detection and screening program. J Am Acad Dermatol 1996;34(6):971–8.

20. US Preventative Services Task Force, Bibbins-Domingo K, Grossman DC, et al. Screening for skin cancer: US Preventative Services Task Force recommendation statement. JAMA 2016;316(4): 429–35.

21. Welch HG, Woloshin S, Schwartz LM. Skin biopsy rates and incidence of melanoma: a population based ecological study. BMJ 2005;331(7515):481.

22. Swerlick RA, Chen S. The melanoma epidemic: more apparent than real? Mayo Clin Proc 1997; 72(6):559–64.

23. Rhodes AR. Intervention strategy to prevent lethal cutaneous melanoma: use of dermatologic photography to aid surveillance of high-risk persons. J Am Acad Dermatol 1998;39(2 Pt 1):262–7.

24. Kelly JW, Yeatman JM, Regalia C, et al. A high incidence of melanoma found in patients with multiple dysplastic naevi by photographic surveillance. Med J Aust 1997;167(4):191–4.

25. Feit NE, Dusza SW, Marghoob AA, et al. Melanomas detected with the aid of total cutaneous photography. Br J Dermatol 2004;150(4):706–14.

26. Goodson AG, Florell SR, Hyde M, et al. Comparative analysis of total body and dermatoscopic photographic monitoring of nevi in similar patient populations at risk for cutaneous melanoma. Dermatol Surg 2010;36(7):1087–98.

27. Tromme I, Sacre L, Hammouch F, et al. Availability of digital dermoscopy in daily practice dramatically reduces the number of excised melanocytic lesions; results from an observational study. Br J Dermatol 2012;167(4):778–86.

28. Gandini S, Sera F, Cattaruzza MS, et al. Meta-analysis of risk factors for cutaneous melanoma: I. Common and atypical naevi. Eur J Cancer 2005;41(1): 28–44.

29. Schiffner R, Schiffner-Rohe J, Landthaler M, et al. Long-term dermoscopic follow-up of melanocytic naevi: clinical outcome and patient compliance. Br J Dermatol 2003;149(1):79–86.

30. Moloney FJ, Guitera P, Coates E, et al. Detection of primary melanoma in individuals at extreme high risk: a prospective 5-year follow-up study. JAMA Dermatol 2014;150(8):819–27.

31. Oliveria SA, Chau D, Christos PJ, et al. Diagnostic accuracy of patients in performing skin self-examination and the impact of photography. Arch Dermatol 2004;140(1):57–62.

32. Moye MS, King SMC, Rice ZP, et al. Effects of total-body digital photography on cancer worry in patients with atypical mole syndrome. JAMA Dermatol 2015;151(2):137–43.

33. Tromme I, Devleesschauwer B, Beutels P, et al. Selective use of sequential digital dermoscopy imaging allows a cost reduction in the melanoma detection process: a Belgian study of patients with a single or a small number of atypical nevi. PLoS One 2014;9(10):e109339.

34. Terushkin V, Oliveria SA, Marghoob AA, et al. Use of and beliefs about total body photography and dermatoscopy among US dermatology training programs: an update. J Am Acad Dermatol 2010; 62(5):794–803.

35. Rice ZP, Weiss FJ, DeLong LK, et al. Utilization and rationale for the implementation of total body (digital) photography as an adjunct screening measure for melanoma. Melanoma Res 2010;20(5):417–21.

36. Murzaku EC, Hayan S, Rao BK. Methods and rates of dermoscopy usage: a cross-sectional survey of US dermatologists stratified by years in practice. J Am Acad Dermatol 2014;71(4):393–5.

37. The Skin Surveillance Process. MoleSafe Web site. Available at: http://molesafe.com/our-services/the-process-ssp/. Accessed November 17, 2016.

38. Foster R. 3-D photography helps early detection in patients at high risk for melanoma. 2015. Available at: https://www.mskcc.org/blog/3-d-photography-helps-early-detection-patients-high-risk-melanoma. Accessed November 15, 2016.

39. Menzies SW, Emery J, Staples M, et al. Impact of dermoscopy and short-term sequential digital dermoscopy imaging for the management of pigmented lesions in primary care: a sequential intervention trial. Br J Dermatol 2009;161(6):1270–7.

40. Zalaudek I, Kittler H, Marghoob AA, et al. Time required for a complete skin examination with and without dermoscopy: a prospective, randomized multicenter study. Arch Dermatol 2008;144(4):509–13.

41. Janda M, Loescher LJ, Banan P, et al. Lesion selection by melanoma high-risk consumers during skin self-examination using mobile teledermoscopy. JAMA Dermatol 2014;150(6):656–8.

42. Mole Mapper. OHSU Dermatology Web site. Available at: https://www.ohsu.edu/xd/health/services/ dermatology/war-on-melanoma/mole-mapper.cfm. Accessed November 17, 2016.

43. Manahan MN, Soyer HP, Loescher LJ, et al. A pilot trial of mobile, patient-performed teledermoscopy. Br J Dermatol 2015;172(4):1072–80.

44. Horsham C, Loescher LJ, Whiteman DC, et al. Consumer acceptance of patient-performed mobile teledermoscopy for the early detection of melanoma. Br J Dermatol 2016;175(6): 1301–10.

# Temporal Image Comparison (Serial Imaging) in Assessing Pigmented Lesions

Rhett J. Drugge, MD[a],*, Elizabeth D. Drugge, PhD, MPH[b]

## KEYWORDS

- Melanoma • Screening • Serial imaging • Two-step method of digital follow-up
- Total body photography • Temporal image comparison

## KEY POINTS

- Lesion evolution is a cardinal sign of cutaneous melanoma (CM).
- Visual skin examination is relatively insensitive to CM, especially small lesions.
- Serial total body photography is sensitive but not specific to CM.
- Short-term serial digital dermatoscopy imaging evolution is specific to CM.

## INTRODUCTION

A slow and inexorable increase in the incidence and mortality of cutaneous melanoma in the United States has been noted since 1935. Albeit small initially, it is a deadly cancer that evades traditional methods of detection. Now, in 2016, more than 10,000 people are projected to succumb to melanoma in the United States.[1]

Limited epidemiologic evidence suggests that the traditional method of melanoma screening is better than oncology treatments for the reduction of melanoma mortality. Studies have shown that the addition of a dermatologist (screening level) service in underserved areas led to a 53% decrease in melanoma mortality, whereas adding a hospital with an oncology department led to a mere 1.9% decrease in melanoma mortality.[2] However, there is insufficient evidence to suggest visual skin examination (VSE) for melanoma screening. Studies demonstrated a lack of sensitivity to melanoma in the hands of dermatologists and primary care physicians alike.[3] New pathways for improved screening merit consideration.

There is a general trend away from comprehensive physical examination for lack of efficacy.[4] Although most melanoma patients have had at least 1 medical visit in the year before their melanoma diagnosis, only 20% reported receiving a skin cancer examination during the melanoma discovery visit.[5] More important, VSE has limited sensitivity. Dermatologists are more sensitive and specific using VSE to detect melanoma than primary care physicians, with a sensitivity and a specificity 49% versus 40% and 97% versus 86%.[6,7] VSE sensitivity to small melanomas ($\leq$3 mm) is very limited; only 2.5% of melanomas are below that threshold.[8] VSE with or without dermoscopy may be performed in less than 3 minutes.[2] Perhaps if melanoma screening were more sensitive to the presence of disease and incorporated into a general physical examination the epidemic would abate.

Disclosure: R.J. Drugge is the inventor of the Melanoscan system, US Patent #7,359,748 and owner of Melanoscan, LLC.
[a] Sheard & Drugge, PC, Stamford Hospital, 30 Shelburne Road, Stamford, CT 06902, USA; [b] Department of Epidemiology and Community Health, New York Medical College School of Health Sciences and Practice, 40 Sunshine Cottage Road, Valhalla, NY 10595, USA
* Corresponding author.
E-mail address: Rhett.drugge@gmail.com

Efforts to screen with greater sensitivity such as with total body photography are currently limited to a small, high-risk population. Furthermore, melanoma screening is generally not offered to those not considered to be at high risk.[9,10] Despite the availability of reimbursement for novel melanoma screening technologies,[11] it has not taken off.

## CUTANEOUS MELANOMA EVOLUTION

The most common presenting cutaneous melanoma (CM) symptom (51%) is an "increase in size."[12] CM arises from melanocytes in the basal epidermal layer,[13] visible to the human eye. The detection of CMs of minute size depends on the observation of abrupt changes most easily detected through comparison of serial imaging, revealing a lesion as small as 1.5 mm.[14] Moreover, small lesions, 1.6 mm diameter, can also be invasive.[15]

CMs grow more rapidly than nevi in a 6- to 12-week period of follow-up.[16] Other monitoring studies documenting observable changes in CMs over a period of months led to the addition of the letter "E" for "evolving" to the ABCD acronym to increase its sensitivity and specificity.[17,18]

Unfortunately, change is obscured by the complex skin patterns of high-risk patients who have too many candidate lesions for human memory to record without imagery. For instance, most young people with melanoma under 40 years of age have an enhanced burden (>25) of nevomelanocytic lesions.[19–21] Those older than 50 years at high risk have severe sun damage,[22] rendering a pattern of autumn leaves on a lawn. Highly reproducible serial imaging is required for sensitive melanoma screening in patients with these common risk factors.

The specificity of change for the diagnosis of CM varies with risk factors. Rates of nevus change are much higher in youth, which decreases the specificity of change as a sign of disease.[23] Conversely, evolution of a mole as a sign specific for CM increases with age.[24] The appearance of new nevi is relatively common even in adults.[25,26] The fact that most CMs arise de novo,[27] and are not contiguously associated with a melanocytic nevus, highlights the importance of imaging the lesion free skin. The specificity of dynamic lesions is further diluted by the exponential increase in keratinocytic lesions with aging.[28] Actinic angiogenesis also contributes to the confusion.[29] Ultraviolet light is the most common carcinogen.[30]

Relatively featureless CMs may be picked up at an early stage by change detection.[31] The most relevant changes associated with CM during sequential digital dermatoscopic imaging (SDDI) are of asymmetric enlargement, an appearance of focal or eccentric new structures (ie, "dermoscopic island"), or the appearance of atypical focal dermoscopic features such as vessels or regression features. Also, CM can appear morphologically more benign over time, at least during short-term monitoring.[32] Melanomas may even be invisible to microscopic inspection.[33]

## SERIAL EVALUATION

Serial image evaluation beyond montage comparison came of age after imagery went digital. Within the past 20 years, skin surface imaging has increasingly emphasized time lapse evaluations. A technique known as SDDI was introduced by colleagues in Austria.[34] In the United States, the total immersion photography (TIP) array, developed in 2000,[35] provided imagery for time lapse tracking over the entire accessible body surface.

Serial total body photography, automated by camera arrays and enhanced by serial dermatoscopy of focal changes, provides a promising sensitivity solution. This highly efficient process, featuring arrays of 25 to 46 cameras, was first introduced as TIP in 2000 with an animated flicker system to harness the eye's motion detection as is done with serial retinal photography.[35] The second step, digital dermatoscopy, was added in 2005 with tracking in 2007.[36,37] Now, the modern 2-step process depends on sequential whole body photography and dermatoscopy (**Fig. 1**) after a baseline examination.

Marino and colleagues[33] have outlined the current best practice for identification and evaluation of new or changing lesions, using TIP, SDDI, and self-examination. Most mapping and tracking camera arrays in use are based on TIP,[35] introduced in 2000, and capable of a variety of applications such as panoramic mosaics of the body, 3-dimensional models of the body, images for use with "machine vision," and interfacing with medical records. One such system, the Melanoscan (Stamford, CT) using TIP, enables users to combine and stack whole body time-series images selected from the patient record to create a sequence where images, total body and dermatoscopic, are scaled, superimposed and flickered. Recently, Canfield (Parsippany, NJ) has introduced a system, WB360 which uses TIP for 3-dimensional display as well. Lesions in TIP systems may be automatically tracked, measured, and compared. Indeed, many mapping and tracking systems are currently available, all with varying degrees of accuracy and efficacy.

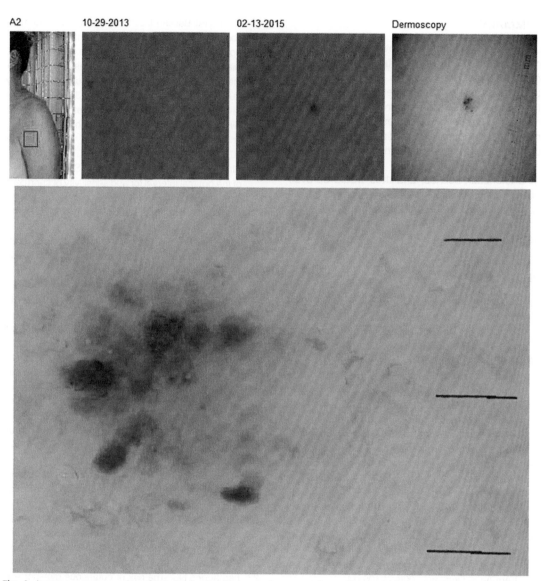

**Fig. 1.** Images accompanying the total body photography report for a 41-year-old woman with no prior history of melanoma. (*Left*) Image captured at the most recent visit. (*Right*) Enlarged images from a previous sessions 1.3 months earlier. (*Far right*) Enlarged image from the captured image on the far left. Semiautomated comparison of images revealed a new melanocytic lesion, less than 2 mm in diameter, which was determined to be an invasive (0.42 mm) melanoma. A dermatoscopy image of the lesion including the dermatoscopic scale, revealed chaos, clods, and amorphous areas.

Over the past 5 years, additional 2-step automated array systems have grown beyond the original Melanoscan system. Arrays have been adopted by several CM-focused groups: the University of Barcelona uses a vertical camera array capturing body images on a turntable[38] and the University of Arizona uses a flat camera array with foot mounts and handlebars for positioning patients.[39] Home-use single camera tracking systems with dermatoscopy have been offered to the public, and although promising, such efforts are hard to evaluate.

## ISSUES TO CONSIDER

Patient compliance is a crucial element to any change detection strategy, and rates of compliance are often lower than desired considering the gravity of the potential diagnosis.[40] Hair, clothing, externally applied pigmentation, mole count, sun damage, and inflammatory skin diseases contribute to false negatives and false positives alike. Limited range of motion, fluctuating body weight, and obesity may also hinder examinations.

## SUMMARY

Large-scale deployment of low-cost, noninvasive mechanisms of early detection are needed to reduce the melanoma burden. A serial 2-step system could power mass screening efforts serving the uninsured and underinsured[41] as well as the rural and remote US counties where melanoma mortality is doubled for lack of access to dermatologists.[2] Furthermore, serial melanoma screening strategies, STBP and SDDI, may be performed as a telehealth service, and thus would be available in any location that can support activity compliant with the Health Insurance Portability and Accountability Act and has appropriate bandwidth.

## REFERENCES

1. Glazer AM, Winkelmann RR, Farberg AS, et al. Analysis of trends in US melanoma incidence and mortality. JAMA Dermatol 2016. http://dx.doi.org/10.1001/jamadermatol.2016.4512.
2. Aneja S, Aneja S, Bordeaux JS. Association of increased dermatologist density with lower melanoma mortality. Arch Dermatol 2012;148:174–8.
3. Wernli KJ, Henrikson NB, Morrison CC, et al. Screening for skin cancer in adults: updated evidence report and systematic review for the us preventive services task force. JAMA 2016;316:436–47.
4. Gøtzsche PC, Jørgensen KJ, Krogsbøll LT. General health checks don't work. BMJ 2014;348:g3680.
5. Koh HK, Miller DR, Geller AC, et al. Who discovers melanoma?: patterns from a population-based survey. J Am Acad Dermatol 1992;26:914–9.
6. Aitken JF, Janda M, Elwood M, et al. Clinical outcomes from skin screening clinics within a community-based melanoma screening program. J Am Acad Dermatol 2006;54:105–14.
7. Fritschi L, Dye SA, Katris P. Validity of melanoma diagnosis in a community-based screening program. Am J Epidemiol 2006;164:385–90.
8. Bono A, Tolomio E, Trincone S, et al. Micro-melanoma detection: a clinical study on 206 consecutive cases of pigmented skin lesions with a diameter ≤ 3 mm. Br J Dermatol 2006;155:570–3.
9. Weinstock MA. Cutaneous melanoma: public health approach to early detection. Dermatol Ther 2006;19: 26–31.
10. Rouhani P, Hu S, Kirsner RS. Melanoma in Hispanic and black Americans. Cancer Control 2008;15: 248–53.
11. Petersen BW, Higgins HW II. Imaging in dermatology. Elsevier; 2016. p. 387–93.
12. Negin BP, Riedel E, Oliveria SA, et al. Symptoms and signs of primary melanoma: important indicators of Breslow depth. Cancer 2003;98:344–8.
13. Shain HA, Bastian BC. From melanocytes to melanomas. Nat Rev Cancer 2016;16:345–58.
14. Rosendahl CO, Drugge ED, Volpicelli ER, et al. Diagnosis of a minute melanoma assisted by automated multi-camera-array total body photography. Australas J Dermatol 2016;57:242–3.
15. Pellizzari G, Magee J, Weedon D, et al. A tiny invasive melanoma: a case report with dermatoscopy and dermatopathology. Dermatol Pract Concept 2013;3:49–51.
16. Altamura D, Avramidis M, Menzies SW. Assessment of the optimal interval for and sensitivity of short-term sequential digital dermoscopy monitoring for the diagnosis of melanoma. Arch Dermatol 2008;144: 502–6.
17. Abbasi NR, Shaw HM, Rigel DS, et al. Early diagnosis of cutaneous melanoma: revisiting the ABCD criteria. JAMA 2004;292:2771–6.
18. American Academy of Dermatology Ad Hoc Task Force for the ABCDEs of Melanoma, Tsao H, Olazagasti JM, Cordoro KM, et al. Early detection of melanoma: reviewing the ABCDEs. J Am Acad Dermatol 2015;72:717–23.
19. Rieger EH, Soyer P, Garbe C, et al. Overall and site-specific risk of malignant melanoma associated with high nevus counts. Melanoma Res 1993;3:36.
20. Taylor NJ, Thomas NE, Anton-Culver H, et al. Nevus count associations with pigmentary phenotype, histopathological melanoma characteristics and survival from melanoma. Int J Cancer 2016;139: 1217–22.
21. Holly EA, Kelly JW, Shpall SN, et al. Number of melanocytic nevi as a major risk factor for malignant melanoma. J Am Acad Dermatol 1987;17:459–68.
22. Gandini S, Sera F, Cattaruzza MS, et al. Meta-analysis of risk factors for cutaneous melanoma: III. Family history, actinic damage and phenotypic factors. Eur J Cancer 2005;41:2040–59.
23. Fernandes NC. The risk of cutaneous melanoma in melanocytic nevi. An Bras Dermatol 2013;88:314–5.
24. Banky JP, Kelly JW, English DR, et al. Incidence of new and changed nevi and melanomas detected using baseline images and dermoscopy in patients at high risk for melanoma. Arch Dermatol 2005; 141:998–1006.
25. Oliveria SA, Yagerman SE, Jaimes N, et al. Clinical and dermoscopic characteristics of new naevi in adults: results from a cohort study. Br J Dermatol 2013;169:848–53.
26. Argenziano G, Cerroni L, Zalaudek I, et al. Accuracy in melanoma detection: a 10-year multicenter survey. J Am Acad Dermatol 2012;67:54–9.
27. Goodson AG, Florell SR, Hyde M, et al. Comparative analysis of total body and dermatoscopic photographic monitoring of nevi in similar patient populations at risk for cutaneous melanoma. Dermatol Surg 2010;36:1087–98.

28. Ortonne JP. Pigmentary changes of the ageing skin. Br J Dermatol 1990;122(Suppl 35):21–8.

29. Chung JH, Eun HC. Angiogenesis in skin aging and photoaging. J Dermatol 2007;34:593–600.

30. Nat Toxicology Program. Report on carcinogens. 12th edition. Diane Publishing; 2011.

31. Kittler H, Guitera P, Riedl E, et al. Identification of clinically featureless incipient melanoma using sequential dermoscopy imaging. Arch Dermatol 2006;142:1113–9.

32. Menzies SW, Gutenev A, Avramidis M, et al. Short-term digital surface microscopic monitoring of atypical or changing melanocytic lesions. Arch Dermatol 2001;137:1583–9.

33. Marino ML, Carrera C, Marchetti MA, et al. Practice Gaps in Dermatology: Melanocytic Lesions and Melanoma. Dermatol Clin 2016;34(3):353–62.

34. Kittler H, Pehamberger H, Wolff K, et al. Follow-up of melanocytic skin lesions with digital epiluminescence microscopy: patterns of modifications observed in early melanoma, atypical nevi, and common nevi. J Am Acad Dermatol 2000;43: 467–76.

35. Drugge R, inventor; Apparatus for total immersion photography. US Patent, 2008.

36. Drugge RJ, Nguyen C, Drugge ED, et al. Melanoma screening with serial whole body photographic change detection using Melanoscan technology. Dermatol Online J 2009;15:1.

37. Drugge RJ, Nguyen C, Gliga L, et al. Clinical pathway for melanoma detection using comprehensive cutaneous analysis with Melanoscan®. Dermatol Online J 2010;16:1.

38. Korotkov K, Quintana J, Puig S, et al. A new total body scanning system for automatic change detection in multiple pigmented skin lesions. IEEE Trans Med Imaging 2015;34:317–38.

39. Seybold K, et al. An automated change detection image analysis system as an aid in the early identification of skin cancer. J Invest Dermatol 2011;131: S130.

40. Madigan LM, Treyger G, Kohen LL. Compliance with serial dermoscopic monitoring: an academic perspective. J Am Acad Dermatol 2016. http://dx.doi.org/10.1016/j.jaad.2016.07.012.

41. Amini A, Rusthoven CG, Waxweiler TV, et al. Association of health insurance with outcomes in adults ages 18 to 64 years with melanoma in the United States. J Am Acad Dermatol 2016; 74:309–16.

# Noninvasive Technologies for the Diagnosis of Cutaneous Melanoma

Richard R. Winkelmann, DO[a],*, Aaron S. Farberg, MD[b],
Alex M. Glazer, MD[c], Darrell S. Rigel, MD, MS[d]

## KEYWORDS

- Melanoma • Technology • Multispectral analysis • Diagnosis • Medical device • Noninvasive

## KEY POINTS

- Multispectral analysis devices assess pigmented lesion disorganization at different levels of the skin using variable wavelengths of light with subsequent computerized analysis.
- Aggregated data investigating the influence of multispectral digital skin lesion analysis on biopsy decisions for melanoma revealed an overall increase in sensitivity from 70% to 88%.
- Five studies using spectrophotometric intracutaneous analysis scope demonstrated an overall sensitivity and specificity of 85% and 81%, respectively, for the detection of melanoma.

## INTRODUCTION

Over the past several decades, there have been many advances in the development of noninvasive technologies that facilitate the early detection of cutaneous melanoma. The use of dermoscopy and total body photography are established modalities proven to enhance the clinical evaluation of pigmented skin lesions at the level of the skin surface. Multispectral analysis devices take advantage of the variable penetration depths of isolated wavelengths of light to assess for pigmented lesion disorganization at different levels of the skin from the surface down to the superficial dermis. Pigmented skin lesion morphology is analyzed via computerized algorithms that measure morphologic disorganization using either melanin alone or in conjunction with hemoglobin and collagen as chromophores.

## CONTENT

Multispectral digital skin lesion analysis (MSDSLA; MelaFind, STRATA Skin Sciences Inc., Horsham, PA) is a medical device that uses visible and near infrared light (430–950 nm) to image pigmented skin lesions at and up to 2.5 mm below the skin surface.[1] Complex computerized analysis uses 75 unique analytical parameters to measure the degree of melanin disorganization within a pigmented skin lesion at 10 different spectral bandwidths. Originally validated on a set of 1432 pigmented lesions with subsequent logistical regression analysis, MSDSLA provides the clinician with the probability the suspicious pigmented skin lesion is a melanoma, and melanoma, high-grade dysplastic nevus, and atypical melanocytic hyperplasia.[2]

Monheit and colleagues[2] used MSDSLA alone to evaluate 1632 suspicious pigmented lesions

Relevant Conflicts of Interest: Drs R.R. Winkelmann, A.S. Farberg and D.S. Rigel served as a consultant to MelaSciences, Inc. Dr A.M. Glazer has no conflicts.

[a] Department of Dermatology, OhioHealth, 40 West Hubbard Avenue, Columbus, OH 43215, USA;
[b] Department of Dermatology, Icahn School of Medicine at Mount Sinai, 5 East 98th Street, New York, NY 10029, USA; [c] National Society for Cutaneous Medicine, 35 East 35th Street #208, New York, NY 10016, USA;
[d] Department of Dermatology, NYU School of Medicine, 35 East 35th Street #208, New York, NY 10016, USA
* Corresponding author.
E-mail address: rrwink@gmail.com

for biopsy, of which 127 were melanoma. The sensitivity of MSDSLA for the detection of melanoma was 98% with a specificity of 11% in recognizing lower risk lesions. In this primarily university-based study, a low disorganization finding was associated with a 98% negative predictive value. However, the frequency and distribution of pigmented lesions that are encountered at high-risk pigmented lesion clinics would be expected to be different than what is experienced in a community-based setting. A subsequent study evaluating the efficacy of MSDSLA in a community-based setting revealed a negative predictive value of 100%.[3]

The influence of MSDSLA on practitioner decisions to biopsy suspicious pigmented skin lesions has been studied in 7 reader studies including 855 practitioners.[4–10] Participants were shown a subset of 62 clinical (distant and close-up) and dermoscopic images of pigmented skin lesions (13 invasive melanomas, 10 melanomas in situ, 7 high-grade dysplastic nevi, and 32 benign skin lesions including low-grade dysplastic nevi) previously analyzed by MSDSLA. Aggregated data revealed the overall sensitivity for the detection of melanoma or other high-grade pigmented lesion improved from 70% after clinical evaluation to 88% after MSDSLA information was provided (P<.001). Participant specificity increased from 52% to 58% (P<.001) after MSDSLA and diagnostic accuracy improved from 59% to 69% (P<.001) with MSDSLA (Table 1).

Spectrophotometric intracutaneous analysis (SIA) scope (SIAscope, Biocompatibles, Farnham, Surrey, UK)[4] was approved by the US Food and Drug Administration in 2011 and also has Health Canada approval and a CE Mark in Europe. The device uses a handheld scanner to measure reflected radiation after exposing the skin to visible and infrared radiation (400–1000 nm). Via computerized algorithms, 8 high-resolution, spectrally filtered color images are analyzed based on total eumelanin, hemoglobin, and collagen content. Studies have found that SIA accurately measures the melanin density across all Fitzpatrick skin types.[5,6]

In an initial study evaluating a set 348 suspicious pigmented skin lesions, SIA had a sensitivity and specificity of 83% and 80%, respectively, for the identification of melanoma.[11] Aggregated data from 5 studies of SIA evaluating suspicious pigmented skin lesions demonstrated an overall sensitivity and specificity of 85% and 81%, respectively, for the detection of 566 melanomas from a total of 4669 pigmented skin lesions (Table 2).

Studies evaluating the use of SIA in the community-based setting have not been as favorable.[14] Govindan and colleagues[7] evaluated the accuracy of general practitioners using SIAscope to refer 886 lesions to a pigmented lesions clinic. The presence of only dermal melanin gave 94.4% sensitivity and 64% specificity for melanoma detection. These data were attributed to the lack of training and negative effects seborrheic keratoses have on the performance of the device.

The original algorithm was modified subsequently to help primary care physicians differentiate seborrheic keratoses and hemangiomas from higher risk pigmented lesions. A new scoring system incorporated the presence of collagen white dots, a cerebriform pattern, blood vessels, and the patient's age into the existing Moncrieff scoring system. The new Molemate system

**Table 1**
**Studies reviewed and aggregated showing impact of MSDSLA on melanoma diagnosis**

| Study, Year | n[a] | Sensitivity (%) | | Specificity (%) | | Biopsy Accuracy (%) | |
| | | Clinical Evaluation | After MSDSLA | Clinical Evaluation | After MSDSLA | Clinical Evaluation | After MSDSLA |
| --- | --- | --- | --- | --- | --- | --- | --- |
| Rigel et al,[9] 2012 | 179 | 69 | 94 | 43 | 25 | — | — |
| Yoo et al,[10] 2013 | 126 | 52 | 77 | 54 | 40 | — | — |
| Winkelmann et al,[11] 2015 | 67 | 67 | 92 | 37 | 57 | 49 | 71 |
| Winkelmann et al,[12] 2015 | 41 | 64 | 62 | 57 | 73 | 60 | 68 |
| Winkelmann et al,[13] 2015 | 212 | 65 | 83 | 40 | 76 | 52 | 80 |
| Winkelmann et al,[14] 2016 | 59 | 59 | 74 | 48 | 56 | 53 | 65 |
| Farberg et al,[15] in press | 160 | 76 | 92 | 52 | 79 | 64 | 86 |
| Aggregate | 855 | 70 | 88 | 52 | 58 | 59 | 69 |

Abbreviation: MDSLA, multispectral digital skin lesion analysis.
  [a] Metaanalysis included all participants in each study including those who did not evaluate the complete set of lesions.

**Table 2**
**Summary of studies evaluating SIA's performance detecting melanoma**

| Study, Year | Number of Lesions | Sensitivity (%) | Specificity (%) |
|---|---|---|---|
| Moncrieff et al,[4] 2002 | 348 | 83 | 80 |
| Haniffa et al,[16] 2007 | 881 | 87 | 91 |
| Glud et al,[17] 2009 | 83 | 100 | 59 |
| Tomatis et al,[18] 2005 | 1391 | 80 | 76 |
| Carrara et al,[19] 2007 | 1966 | 88 | 80 |
| Aggregate | 4669 | 85 | 81 |

*Abbreviation:* SIA, spectrophotometric intracutaneous analysis.

(MMS; Biocompatibles) was studied in a randomized, controlled trial evaluating primary care practitioner biopsy rates in 1297 patients presenting with 1573 nonbenign pigmented skin lesions.[8] Study arms were divided into groups being evaluated with clinical history, naked eye examination, and dermoscopy with or without MMS. The sensitivity for the detection of melanoma in the group using MMS versus best practices only was 100% (18/18) and 94% (17/18), respectively. Interestingly, the percent agreement between primary care practitioner and expert analysis that a lesion was benign was lower using MMS than by best practices alone (84% vs 91%, respectively; $P<.001$).

## DISCUSSION

With growing trends in health care emphasizing the need for efficient and cost-effective medical practice, the routine use of diagnostic technologies to optimize the clinical evaluation of suspicious pigmented skin lesions by dermatologists and other health care providers seems inevitable. The risk of missing a melanoma using multispectral analysis led companies to prioritize high levels of sensitivity for their devices with lower specificity as a consequence. For this reason and other ambiguous practical considerations, like device and patient costs, the implementation of these technologies into routine practice has been indolent. Nonetheless, studies have demonstrated that the use of information provided by the computerized analysis of pigmented skin lesions obtained by multispectral analysis devices provides additional, beneficial clinical data for practitioners to incorporate into their biopsy decisions.

## REFERENCES

1. Elbaum M, Kopf AW, Rabinovitz HS, et al. Automatic differentiation of melanoma and melanocytic nevi with multispectral digital dermoscopy: a feasibility study. J Am Acad Dermatol 2001;44(2):207–18.
2. Monheit G, Cognetta AB, Ferris L, et al. The performance of MelaFind: a prospective multicenter study. Arch Dermatol 2011;147(2):188–94.
3. Winkelmann RR, Rigel DS, Kollmann E, et al. Negative predictive value of pigmented lesion evaluation by multispectral digital skin lesion analysis in a community practice setting. J Clin Aesthet Dermatol 2015;8(3):745–7.
4. Moncrieff M, Cotton S, Claridge E, et al. Spectrophotometric intracutaneous analysis: a new technique for imaging pigmented skin lesions. Br J Dermatol 2002;146:448–57.
5. Claridge E, Cotton S, Hall P, et al. From colour to tissue histology: physics-based interpretation of images of pigmented skin lesions. Med Image Anal 2003;7:489–502.
6. Matts PJ, Dykes PJ, Marks R. The distribution of melanin in skin determined in vivo. Br J Dermatol 2007;156:620–8.
7. Govindan K, Smith J, Knowles L, et al. Assessment of nurse-led screening of pigmented lesions using SIAscope. J Plast Reconstr Aesthet Surg 2007;60: 639–45.
8. Walter FM, Morris HC, Humphrys E, et al. Effect of adding a diagnostic aid to best practice to manage suspicious pigmented lesions in primary care: randomized controlled trial. BMJ 2012;345:e4110.
9. Rigel DS, Roy M, Yoo J, et al. Impact of guidance from a computer-aided multispectral digital skin lesion analysis device on decision to biopsy lesions clinically suggestive of melanoma. Arch Dermatol 2012;148:541–3.
10. Yoo J, Rigel DS, Roy M, et al. Impact of guidance from a multispectral digital skin lesion analysis device on dermatology residents' decisions to biopsy lesions clinically suggestive of melanoma. J Am Acad Dermatol 2013;68(4):AB152.
11. Winkelmann RR, Yoo J, Tucker N, et al. Impact of guidance provided by a multispectral digital skin lesion analysis device following dermoscopy on

decisions to biopsy atypical melanocytic lesions. J Clin Aesthet Dermatol 2015;8(9):21–4.

12. Winkelmann RR, Hauschild A, Tucker N, et al. The impact of multispectral digital skin lesion analysis on German dermatologist decisions to biopsy atypical pigmented lesions with clinical characteristics of melanoma. J Clin Aesthet Dermatol 2015;8(10): 27–9.

13. Winkelmann RR, Tucker N, White R, et al. Pigmented skin lesion biopsies after computer-aided multispectral digital skin lesion analysis. J Am Osteopath Assoc 2015;115(11):666–9.

14. Winkelmann RR, Farberg AS, Tucker N, et al. Enhancement of international dermatologists' pigmented skin lesion biopsy decisions following dermoscopy with subsequent integration of multispectral digital skin lesion analysis. J Clin Aesthet Dermatol 2016;9(7):53–5.

15. Farberg AS, Winkelmann RR, Tucker N, et al. The impact of quantitative data provided by a multispectral digital skin lesion analysis device on

dermatologists' decisions to biopsy pigmented lesions. J Clin Aesthet Dermatol, in press.

16. Haniffa MA, Lloyd JJ, Lawrence CM. The use of a spectrophotometric intracutaneous analysis device in the real-time diagnosis of melanoma in the setting of a melanoma screening clinic. Br J Dermatol 2007; 156:1350–2.

17. Glud M, Gniadecki R, Drzewiecki KT. Spectrophotometric intracutaneous analysis versus dermoscopy for the diagnosis of pigmented skin lesions: prospective, double-blind study in a secondary reference centre. Melanoma Res 2009;19:176–9.

18. Tomatis S, Carrara M, Bono A, et al. Automated melanoma detection with a novel multispectral imaging system: results of a prospective study. Phys Med Biol 2005;50:1675–87.

19. Carrara M, Bono A, Bartoli C, et al. Multispectral imaging and artificial neural network: mimicking the management decision of the clinician facing pigmented skin lesions. Phys Med Biol 2007;52: 2599–613.

# Using Reflectance Confocal Microscopy in Skin Cancer Diagnosis

Attiya Haroon, MD, PhD*, Shahram Shafi, MD,
Babar K. Rao, MD

## KEYWORDS

- Reflectance confocal microscopy • Melanocytic skin cancer • Nonmelanocytic skin cancer

## KEY POINTS

- Reflectance confocal microcopy (RCM) is a noninvasive diagnostic technique that enables visualization of different skin layers at an almost histologic resolution.
- RCM shows distinct confocal features for different skin lesions, which allows benign skin lesions to be successfully differentiated from malignant lesions.
- With further studies and more widespread physician training in the technique, RCM has the potential to revolutionize the field of skin cancer tissue diagnosis.

## INTRODUCTION

Until now, biopsy and histologic evaluation has been the gold standard to diagnose skin tumors. Reflectance confocal microcopy (RCM) is a noninvasive, innovative, and 21st century diagnostic technique that enables visualization of different skin layers at an almost histologic resolution.[1] In the past decade RCM has been proven beneficial in management of various cutaneous lesions.[2] The aim of this article is to highlight the clinical significance and future of RCM to diagnose common skin cancers. Confocal diagnostic features of benign melanocytic nevi, lentigo maligna, melanoma, squamous cell carcinoma (SCC), and basal cell carcinoma (BCC) are discussed in this article.

## PRINCIPLE OF REFLECTANCE CONFOCAL MICROCOPY

The principle of RCM is based on focal point illumination and hence named confocal microscopy. The device uses a low power laser beam (infrared wavelength of 830 nm) to illuminate a small point inside the skin tissue. This light is reflected back through a small pinhole and is imaged on the detector. The pinhole aperture filters the scattered and reflected light and allows only the light from image plane to pass through it.[3] In this way, the computer software produces a high-resolution, 2-dimensional, gray scale image of target lesion. Conventional RCM enables imaging depth up to 200 to 300 μm, which corresponds with the papillary dermis.[4]

## HOW TO PERFORM REFLECTANCE CONFOCAL MICROSCOPY

Fig. 1 displays a US Food and Drug Administration–approved clinical reflectance confocal microscope. Reflectance confocal microscopy is simple and quick procedure. Patient demographics with lesion history are entered into the computer software and the patient is prepared for confocal microscopy. A small drop of oil is applied to the target lesion and a metal ring with polymer or glass window is attached to the skin

Disclosure Statement: Consultant for the caliber ID (maker of Vivascope).
Department of Dermatology, Rutgers-Robert Wood Johnson Medical School, 1 Worlds Fair Drive, 2nd Floor, Suite 2400, Somerset, NJ 08873, USA
* Corresponding author.
E-mail address: Attiya.haroon@gmail.com

derm.theclinics.com

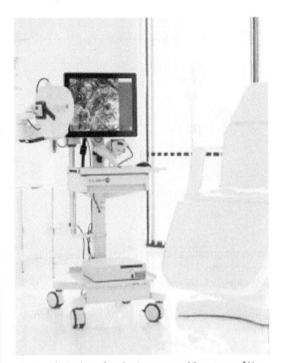

**Fig. 1.** Clinical confocal microscope. (*Courtesy of* Non-Invasive Diagnostic Imaging of the Skin (NIDIskin), New York, NY; with permission.)

with the aid of an adhesive tape. A dermoscopy image is obtained with the vivacam through this metal ring. Next, ultrasound gel with a refractive index close to the epidermis is applied inside the metal ring. The metal ring is then connected magnetically with the vivascope head. RCM images composed of viva cubes and viva stacks are obtained at different skin layers including the epidermis, dermoepidermal junction, and upper dermis. These confocal images are stored and transferred through a high-speed Internet system to the clinical expert for analysis of the confocal images.[5]

## REFLECTANCE CONFOCAL MICROCOPY AND SKIN CANCER DIAGNOSIS

Nonmelanoma skin cancer, including SCC and BCC, constitutes the most common cancers in the United States. Melanoma skin cancer—although not the most common—has a notably higher mortality, rate causing more than 75% of all skin cancer deaths. However, early detection and better management can improve the prognosis of melanoma patients. With the aid of reflectance confocal microscopy, benign skin lesions can be differentiated successfully from malignant lesions. RCM shows distinct confocal features for different skin lesions.[6] These confocal features

aid in quick bedside diagnosis of melanoma and nonmelanoma skin cancers.[7]

## MELANOCYTIC CANCER DIAGNOSIS

To recognize confocal features of melanocytic cancer, we must first revise the features of benign melanocytic lesions such as benign melanocytic nevi (**Table 1**). Benign melanocytic nevi has symmetric architecture, well-circumscribed regular honeycomb or cobblestone pattern of the epidermis, edged papillae, and homogenous dense and sparse dermal nests (**Fig. 2**)[1,6,8]

### Lentigo Maligna

It is difficult to differentiate clinically between lentigo simplex and lentigo maligna, which is the

**Table 1**
**Characteristic confocal features of melanocytic skin tumors**

| Type of Melanocytic Tumors | Characteristic Confocal Features |
|---|---|
| Benign melanocytic nevus | Symmetric architecture. *Epidermis*: Honeycomb or cobblestone pattern. *DEJ*: Regular ring pattern, edged or nonedged papillae. *Dermis*: Homogenous dense and sparse dermal nests. |
| Lentigo maligna | *Epidermis*: Disruption of the typical honeycomb or cobblestone pattern. Multiple large round pagetoid cells. *DEJ*: Disorganized architecture, nonedged papillae, atypical pleomorphic cells. *Dermis*: Large nucleated cells, plump bright cells |
| Malignant melanoma | *Epidermis*: Irregular honeycomb or cobblestone pattern, large nucleated pagetoid cells. *DEJ*: Disorganized ringed, meshwork, or unspecific pattern. Edged or nonedged papillae, uneven clusters and single atypical cells. *Dermis*: Dense and sparse nests of cells, plump bright and small bright cells, increased reticulated, curled and fragmented bright collagen fibers. |

*Abbreviation:* DEJ, dermoepidermal junction.

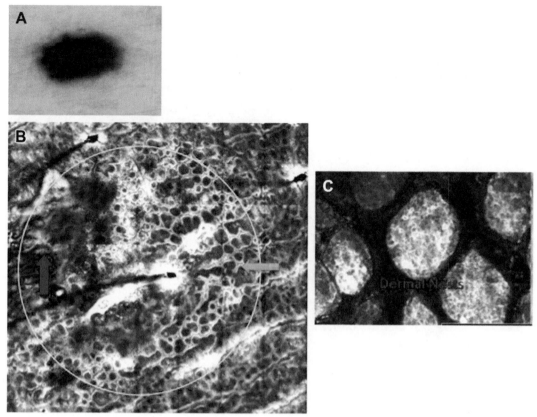

**Fig. 2.** (*A*) Dermoscopy image shows a lesion with the regular pigment network. (*B*) Confocal microscopy image shows regular honeycomb pattern, ringed edged papillae (*blue arrow*), and dermal nests (*red arrow*). These features are characteristic of benign melanocytic nevus. (*C*) High-resolution confocal image showing dermal nests.

most common type of facial melanoma.[9] RCM not only helps to make the right diagnosis, but also prevents the patients from having an unnecessary scar in case of a benign lesion on esthetically significant site. In the case of a large-sized lentigo, where a biopsy is taken from only a small area, a physician can miss a cancer diagnosis. RCM is beneficial in that the entire lesion may be imaged, enabling the physician to better diagnose a lesion.

Confocal features of lentigo maligna include disruption of the typical honeycomb or cobblestone pattern of the epidermis and the presence of multiple round pagetoid cells.[1] The dermoepidermal junction shows a disorganized architecture and nonedged papillae. There are atypical pleomorphic cells defined as reflective cells with a size more than twice the diameter of keratinocytes. These cells have irregular shapes. Large nucleated cells may be seen within the dermal papillae.[1]

## Melanoma

Approximately 1.9% of men and women will be diagnosed with invasive melanoma at some point

during their lifetime.[10] The prognosis of melanoma depends largely on early diagnosis and timely management. RCM has revolutionized the management of melanoma by enabling physicians to make a quick bedside diagnosis.[11] RCM features of melanoma have been well-studied and described in the last decade. Confocal features of melanoma includes irregular honeycomb or cobblestone pattern in the epidermis. The dermoepidermal junction shows complete architectural disarrangements with edged and nonedged papillae and cells with a size twice the size of keratinocytes[1] (**Fig. 3**). Large, round, nucleated cells with irregular shapes called pagetoid cells are also seen in melanomas.

Pellacani and colleagues[12] did an extensive study including 16,618 pigmented skin lesions and designed a diagnostic model for melanoma. This model requires identification of 6 confocal features, 2 major and 4 minor. The presence of 1 major and 1 minor criterion is essential for the diagnosis of melanoma. The 2 major criteria include the presence of cytologic atypia and nonedged papillae at the basal layer. The 4 minor

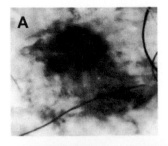

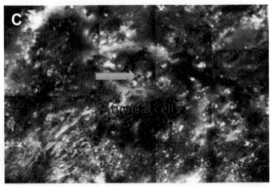

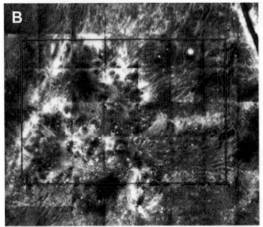

Fig. 3. (*A*) Dermoscopy image shows a lesion with irregular pigment network and multiple colors. (*B*) Confocal microscopy image shows nonedged papillae, uneven clusters of atypical cells, and pagetoid cells infiltration (*red square*). These features are characteristic of melanoma. (*C*) High-resolution confocal image showing atypical cells (*blue arrow*).

criteria include round cells in the superficial layers, pagetoid cells throughout the lesion, cerebriform clusters in the papillary dermis, and nucleated cells within the dermal papilla.

***Diagnostic accuracy of melanocytic skin cancer diagnosis using reflectance confocal microcopy***
The analysis of sensitivity and specificity of melanocytic skin cancer diagnosis using RCM is crucial to have a clear picture about the clinical application of RCM.

Pellacani and colleagues[13] analyzed 351 melanocytic lesions (malignant melanoma, melanoma in situ, melanocytic nevi) from 332 patients to assess diagnostic accuracy. The study reported a sensitivity of 92% and specificity of 69%.

Rao and colleagues[14] in a recent retrospective study analyzed 748 clinically suspicious lesions. Of these, 629 lesions displayed benign features on confocal and hence did not require a biopsy. For remaining 119 lesions where a subsequent biopsy was done, a confocal and histopathologic comparison was done. A sensitivity of 100% and specificity of 92.6% was reported. The author attributed this high rate of diagnostic accuracy to

his experience gained using RCM in his clinical practice.

## NONMELANOCYTIC SKIN CANCER DIAGNOSIS

Table 2 summarizes the confocal features of nonmelanocytic skin tumors.

### Basal Cell Carcinoma

The most common sites of BCC are the face, nose, and eyelids. Dermsocopy has a high positive predictive value for diagnosis of BCC. The addition of RCM could potentially increase the sensitivity of diagnosis of BCC.[15] Additionally, RCM could also help the surgeon to decide about the size and margins to be removed in case of a malignant lesion.

Confocal features of BCC include islands of tumor cells with elongated nuclei orientated at the same axis, a phenomenon known as *polarization* of nuclei, and *clefting*, the separation of tumor islands from the surrounding stroma (**Fig. 4**). This clefting noticed on RCM is probably because of mucin deposits seen on histology.[16] The epidermis

| Table 2 Characteristic confocal features of nonmelanocytic skin tumors | |
|---|---|
| Type of Nonmelanocytic Skin Tumor | Characteristic Confocal Features |
| Basal cell carcinoma | Bright, round to oval lobulated tumor islands in DEJ, dark silhouette spaces, nuclei polarization of the tumor cells along the same axis (streaming), thick tortuous vessels and small bright inflammatory cells. |
| Actinic keratosis | Hyperkeratosis, parakeratosis, atypical honeycomb or cobblestone pattern of epidermis with uneven dysplastic keratinocytes and irregular cell borders. Solar elastosis in dermis. |
| Squamous cell carcinoma | Hyperkeratosis, parakeratosis, atypical honeycomb or disarranged pattern with uneven dysplastic detached keratinocytes and irregular cell outlines. Round nucleated and dendritic bright cells infiltrating the dermis. Round vessels parallel to dermal papillae. |

Abbreviation: DEJ, dermoepidermal junction.

shows an irregular honeycomb or cobblestone pattern above tumor islands. The dark silhouette sign is also a characteristic RCM feature of BCC. Telangiectasia is a clinical feature of BCC, which is seen as an increase in the number and size of round spaces containing moving blood cells on RCM.[1] Nori and colleagues[17] did an extensive study on confocal features of BCC with 152 skin lesions from 4 institutions. They found a 100% sensitivity for BCC diagnosis with RCM with the presence of 2 or more criteria.

Kadouch and colleagues[18] performed a meta-analysis on the accuracy of diagnosis of BCC using RCM. The study concluded a sensitivity and specificity of 95% each. Despite the high sensitivity and specificity, more studies are required to draw a firm conclusion about the accuracy of RCM diagnosis of BCC.

BCC has various histologic types, including superficial, nodular, pigmented, and morpheaform. Although a general criterion has been established for RCM diagnosis of BCC, recent studies have shown a histologic–confocal correlation between different variants of BCC.[19] Proliferation and atypia of dendritic cells are features of melanoma; however, benign dendritic cells have been seen in pigmented BCC. Segura and colleagues[20] reported the presence of highly refractile dendritic structures corresponding with melanocytes and Langerhans cells on RCM.

## Actinic Keratosis

Actinic keratosis (AK) is a common nonmelanocytic skin lesion, especially seen among fair skinned and elderly people. AK is an atypical proliferation of epidermal keratinocytes. The tendency of AK to transform into SCC warrants a continuous monitoring of this skin lesion. Histologic examination is the gold standard for AK diagnosis; however, RCM has the potential to differentiate AK from SCC. According to atlas of confocal microscopy by Rao and colleagues,[1] the epidermis shows parakeratosis and hyperkeratosis on RCM in AK. There is an atypical honeycomb pattern with uneven dysplastic keratinocytes (Fig. 5). RCM images of the dermis show signs of solar elastosis with moderately refractive lacelike material adjacent to the collagen bundle.

Ulrich and colleagues[21,22] studied 44 patients diagnosed with AK using the confocal microscope. They concluded that architectural disarray and cellular pleomorphism were the best indicators of AK confocally. The sensitivity and specificity of AK diagnosis with RCM was 80% to 98%.

## Squamous Cell Carcinoma

SCC usually occurs on sun-exposed areas like the head, neck, and back of the hands. About 700,000 new cases of SCC are diagnosed each year in United States. Bowen disease is SCC in situ, which could be confused clinically with certain inflammatory or nonmelanoma skin tumors. According to a recent review by Ulrich and colleagues,[23] RCM features of Bowen disease are the disruption of stratum corneum and atypical honeycomb pattern of the epidermis. Dyskeratotic cells are also seen. Dark circular spaces in the center of the papillary rings and S-shaped blood vessels are also signs of Bowen disease.

RCM images of SCC show hyperkeratosis and parakeratosis of the stratum corneum. An atypical honeycomb pattern with uneven dysplastic cells, detached keratinocytes, and irregular cell outlines are characteristic RCM features of SCC (Fig. 6). Round, nucleated, and dendritic bright single cells infiltrating the dermis are also seen in SCC. The dermoepidermal junction shows edged and nonedged papillae.[1,24]

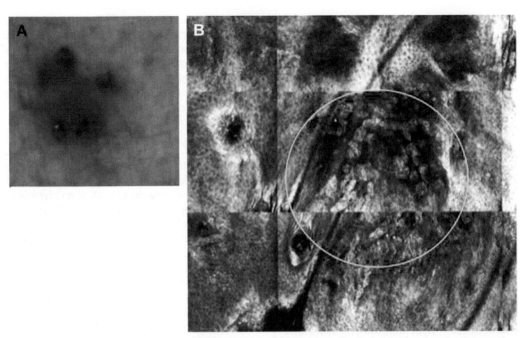

**Fig. 4.** (*A*) Dermoscopy image shows an ovoid brownish erythematous flat lesion with telangiectasia at the periphery of the lesion. (*B*) Confocal microscopy image shows islands of tumor cells (*yellow circle*). Tumor cells are large, irregular, and have elongated nuclei with peripheral palisading. These cells are separated by dark cleft-like spaces.

### Limitations of the technique

RCM can image the skin lesion up to 250 to 300 μm and hence only those lesions limited to the upper dermis can be diagnosed on RCM.

Also, for the analysis of confocal images, few trained physicians are available. This emphasizes the importance of generating more awareness about RCM among physicians.

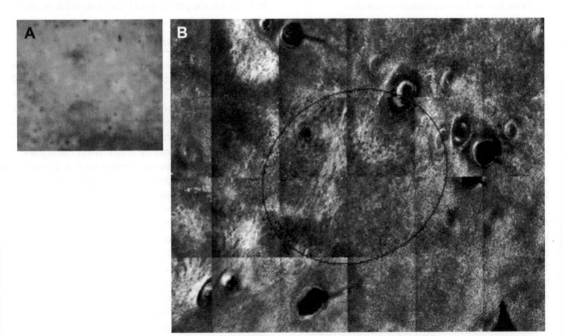

**Fig. 5.** (*A*) Dermoscopy image shows brownish erythematous plaque with central scaling. (*B*) Confocal images show hyperkeratosis and irregular honeycomb pattern of epidermis and dysplastic keratinocytes (*red oval*). These features are characteristic of actinic keratosis.

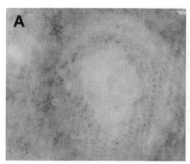
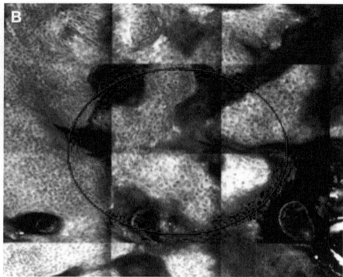

**Fig. 6.** (*A*) Dermoscopy image shows erythematous lesion with strawberry-shaped vessels at the border. (*B*) Confocal images show atypical honeycomb pattern (*red circle*), detached keratinocytes, and irregular cell outlines. These features are characteristic of squamous cell carcinoma.

## SUMMARY

Although RCM has a potential to revolutionize the field of skin cancer tissue diagnosis, currently RCM cannot replace standard histopathologic diagnosis. More studies are required to better compare the sensitivity and specificity of skin cancer diagnosis using RCM.

## REFERENCES

1. BK. Rao. Atlas of confocal microscopy in dermatology. NIDISkin; 2013, ISBN 978–0578119953.

2. Fink C, Haenssle HA. Non-invasive tools for the diagnosis of cutaneous melanoma. Skin Res Technol 2016. http://dx.doi.org/10.1111/srt.12350.

3. Que SKT, Fraga-Braghiroli N, Grant-Kels JM, et al. Through the looking glass: Basics and principles of reflectance confocal microscopy. J Am Acad Dermatol 2015;73:276–84.

4. Batta MM, Kessler ES, White PF. Reflectance confocal microscopy: An overview of technology and advances in telepathology. Cutis 2015;95: 39–46.

5. Calzavara-Pinton P, Longo C, Venturini M. Reflectance confocal microscopy for in vivo skin imaging. Photochem Photobiol 2008;84:1421–30.

6. Hofmann-Wellenhoff R, Pellacani G, Malvehy, J, et al. Reflectance confocal microscopy for skin diseases. Springer; 2012 ISBN 978-3-642-21997-9.

7. Scope A, Benvenuto-Andrade C, Agero AC, et al. In vivo reflectance confocal microscopy imaging of melanocytic skin lesions: consensus terminology glossary and illustrative images. J Am Acad Dermatol 2007;57:644–58.

8. Scope A, Benvenuto-Andrade C, Agero AL, et al. Correlation of dermoscopic structures of melanocytic lesions to reflectance confocal microscopy. Arch Dermatol 2007;143:176–85.

9. Gamo R, Pampín A, Floristán U. Reflectance confocal microscopy in lentigo maligna. Actas Dermosifiliogr 2016;107:830–5.

10. Glazer AM, Winkelmann RR, Farberg AS, et al. Analysis of trends in US melanoma incidence and mortality. JAMA Dermatol 2016. http://dx.doi.org/10.1001/jamadermatol.2016.4512.

11. Pellacani G, Farnetani F, Gonzalez S, et al. In vivo confocal microscopy for detection and grading of dysplastic nevi: a pilot study. J Am Acad Dermatol 2012;66(3):e109–21.

12. Pellacani G, Cesinaro AM, Seidenari S. Reflectance confocal microscopy of pigmented skin lesions:-improvement in melanoma diagnostic specificity. J Am Acad Dermatol 2005;53:977–85.

13. Pellacani G, Guitera P, Longo C, et al. The impact of in vivo reflectance confocal microscopy for the diagnostic accuracy of melanoma and equivocal melanocytic lesions. J Invest Dermatol 2007;27:59–65.

14. Giambrone D, Alamgir M, Masud A, et al. The diagnostic accuracy of in vivo confocal microscopy in clinical practice. J Am Acad Dermatol 2015;73: 317–9.

15. Ulrich M, Lange-Asschenfeldt S, González S, et al. In vivo reflectance confocal microscopy for early diagnosis of nonmelanoma skin cancer. Actas Dermosifiliogr 2012;103:784–9.

16. González S, Sánchez V, González-Rodríguez A, et al. Confocal microscopy patterns in non melanoma skin cancer and clinical applications. Actas Dermosifiliogr 2014;152(2):169–77.

17. Nori S, Rius-Díaz F, Cuevas J, et al. Sensitivity and specificity of reflectance-mode confocal microscopy for in vivo diagnosis of basal cell carcinoma: a multicenter study. J Am Acad Dermatol 2004;51: 923–30.

18. Kadouch DJ, Schram ME, Leeflang MM, et al. In vivo reflectance confocal microscopy of basal cell carcinoma: a systemic review of diagnostic accuracy. J Eur Acad Dermatol Venereol 2015;29: 1890–7.

19. Agero AL, Busam KJ, Benvenuto-Andrade C, et al. Reflectance confocal microscopy of pigmented basal cell carcinoma. J Am Acad Dermatol 2006; 54(4):638–43.

20. Segura S, Puig S, Carrera C, et al. Dendritic cells in pigmented basal cell carcinoma: a relevant finding by reflectance-mode confocal microscopy. Arch Dermatol 2007;143:883–6.

21. Ulrich M, Maltusch A, Rius-Diaz F, et al. Clinical applicability of in vivo reflectance confocal microscopy for the diagnosis of actinic keratoses. Dermatol Surg 2008;34:610–9.

22. Ulrich M, Maltusch A, Röwert-Huber J, et al. Actinic keratoses: non-invasive diagnosis for field cancerisation. Br J Dermatol 2007;156:13–7.

23. Ulrich M, Kanitakis J, González S, et al. Evaluation of Bowen disease by in vivo reflectance confocal microscopy. Br J Dermatol 2012;166:451–3.

24. Rishpon A, Kim N, Scope A, et al. Reflectance confocal microscopy criteria for squamous cell carcinomas and actinic keratosis. Arch Dermatol 2009;145:766–72.

# Optical Coherence Tomography in the Diagnosis of Skin Cancer

Amanda Levine, MD[a,b,c], Katie Wang, DO[a,b,c],
Orit Markowitz, MD[a,b,c],*

## KEYWORDS

- Optical coherence tomography • Nonmelanoma skin cancer • Melanoma • Noninvasive imaging

## KEY POINTS

- A review of the literature shows that optical coherence tomography (OCT) increases the overall sensitivity, specificity, and diagnostic accuracy compared with clinical and dermoscopy evaluation alone.
- Frequency Domain OCT (FD-OCT) has imaging depth of up to 2 mm, with enough cellular clarity to diagnose nonmelanoma skin cancers. Dynamic OCT (D-OCT) enables us to visualize vascular patterns in the skin, improving diagnostic accuracy. Finally, high-definition OCT (HD-OCT) has improved cellular resolution compared with FD-OCT and D-OCT, at the sacrifice of penetration depth and field of view. However, HD-OCT serves to fill the gap between reflectance confocal microscopy and conventional FD-OCT.
- OCT has also been shown to be useful in tumor margin delineation and is, thus, useful in preoperative treatment planning. In addition, OCT enables noninvasive treatment monitoring of skin cancers undergoing nonsurgical therapies.

## INTRODUCTION

Over the past decade, optical coherence tomography (OCT) has emerged as a novel noninvasive imaging device that allows for the real-time, in vivo, cross-sectional imaging of skin morphology. The advantage of these noninvasive devices over histopathology is that they enable repeated imaging of the same unaltered skin sites to observe dynamic events and long-term changes over time. Therefore, OCT has been used in both clinical and research settings to aid in the diagnosis of clinical and subclinical lesions; delineate lesion margins; and, unique to OCT given its larger field of view

(FOV) and increased depth, monitor lesions undergoing nonsurgical treatment.

## OPTICAL COHERENCE TOMOGRAPHY

OCT imaging is based on low-coherence interferometry to detect the intensity of backscattered infrared light from biological tissues by measuring the optical path length.[1–4] With these imaging devices, there is an inverse relationship between cellular clarity and both FOV as well as depth.[1] Basically, as imaging depth and lateral resolution increases, the cellular resolution decreases (Table 1).

Disclosure Statement: Dr O. Markowitz is an investigator for Michelson Diagnostics and Caliber ID. Dr A. Levine and Dr K. Wang have nothing to disclose.
[a] Department of Dermatology, SUNY Downstate Medical Center, 450 Clarkson Avenue, Brooklyn, NY 11203, USA; [b] Department of Dermatology, VA NY Harbor Health Care System, 800 Poly Place, Brooklyn, NY 11209, USA; [c] Department of Dermatology, Mount Sinai Medical Center, 5 East 98th Street, New York, NY 10029, USA
* Corresponding author. 5 East 98th Street, New York, NY 10029.
E-mail address: omarkowitz@gmail.com

Dermatol Clin 35 (2017) 465–488
http://dx.doi.org/10.1016/j.det.2017.06.008

**Table 1**
**Summary of noninvasive imaging devices**

| Imaging Modality | Imaging Depth (mm) | Lateral Resolution (μm) | Axial Resolution (μm) | FOV (mm) | Probe Aperture Size |
|---|---|---|---|---|---|
| RCM | 0.2 | 0.5–1.0 | 3–5 | 0.5 × 0.5 | 3.16 cm |
| HD-OCT | 0.57 | 3 | 3 | 1.8 × 1.5 | 5 cm |
| FD-OCT, D-OCT/ SV-OCT | 1.5–2.0 | 7.5 | 5 | 6.0 × 6.0 | 1.38 cm |
| HFUS (20 MHz) | 10 | 200 | 80 | 12 | 10–20 mm |

*Abbreviations:* D-OCT, dynamic OCT; FD-OCT, Frequency Domain OCT; HD-OCT, high-definition OCT; HFUS, high-frequency ultrasound; RCM, reflectance confocal microscopy; SV-OCT, speckle variance OCT.

There are several different OCT imaging modalities that have been studied. The swept-source multi-beam Frequency Domain OCT (FD-OCT) (Vivosight, Michelson Diagnostics, Kent, United Kingdom) provides 2 real-time imaging modes: b-scan (vertical, cross-sectional), similar to histology, and en face modes (horizontal), similar to that of dermoscopy and reflectance confocal microscopy (RCM). The images have an optical resolution of less than 7.5 μm laterally and less than 5 μm axially, a penetration depth of up to 2 mm, and an FOV of 6.0 mm × 6.0 mm.[1–4] A recent advancement, dynamic OCT (D-OCT) based on speckle variance OCT (SV-OCT), allows for visualization of skin microvasculature and the detection of blood flow.[1] Angiogenesis is important in the growth and spread of cancers; thus, visualization of vessel morphology is helpful in improving diagnostic accuracy.

Although conventional FD-OCT has been shown to be useful in skin imaging, its limited resolution precludes visualization of the skin at the cellular level. High-definition OCT (HD-OCT) (Skintell device, Agfa Healthcare, Mortsel, Belgium) seems to bridge the gap between conventional FD-OCT imaging and RCM offering improved axial and lateral resolution of 3 μm, with the trade-off of a more limited penetration depth of about 750 μm and FOV of 1.8 mm × 1.5 mm.[1–4]

High-frequency ultrasound is another imaging modality that has the largest penetration depth and FOV, however, lacks the cellular resolution necessary for skin visualization (<1 mm) and is, therefore, not frequently used in the diagnosis and management of skin.[5]

When comparing the different imaging methods, it is important to be aware of the imaging mode. FD-OCT, D-OCT, and HD-OCT devices all provide both vertical and horizontal en face images, creating a 3-dimensional image.[2–4] The vertical scans are helpful in that they mimic histology sections; the horizontal view, similar to RCM, helps bridge the gap of dermoscopy to histology.

Another parameter to consider is the probe aperture size to FOV ratio. Noninvasive devices have a probe that directly touches the skin and produces an image based on its FOV. Usually the FOV is much smaller than the probe itself. The smaller the aperture and the larger the FOV the less of a discrepancy between what the probe comes in contact with and what is actually being imaged. Thus, a smaller variation in the aperture to FOV ratio leads to more accurate probe placement and, therefore, a better correlation of what you are imaging and what you see clinically. This smaller variation is especially important at varying time points if, for example, you are monitoring a lesion undergoing treatment. Additionally, a small probe can be positioned to image in more cosmetically sensitive areas, such as the head and neck. Ultrasound has the best FOV to aperture size ratio followed by FD- and D-OCT as seen in **Table 1**.

## FREQUENCY DOMAIN-OPTICAL COHERENCE TOMOGRAPHY

FD-OCT has mainly been used in the cross-sectional (vertical mode) similar to histology (**Table 2**).

### Basal Cell Carcinoma

There have been several studies investigating the accuracy of FD-OCT in diagnosis of basal cell carcinoma (BCC). The literature indicates that FD-OCT increased sensitivity, specificity, and diagnostic accuracy compared with clinical and dermoscopy assessment alone.[6–11] There are few studies showing that FD-OCT is able to distinguish between the different BCC subtypes.[7–9] However, some studies think FD-OCT lacks the cellular clarity to make this distinction.

The major diagnostic criteria on FD-OCT for BCC are alteration of the dermoepidermal junction (DEJ) and dark ovoid basal cell islands in the dermis, which are typically surrounded by a darker, hyporeflective peripheral border.[6–11] Often

**Table 2**
Frequency Domain

| First Author, Year, Country | Population Characteristics | Lesions, Number | Accuracy | Findings/Results | Limitations |
|---|---|---|---|---|---|
| Maher et al,[28] 2016, Australia | 88 patients (47 M, 28 F), mean age 63 y | 88 equivocal amelanotic or hypomelanotic skin lesions (AHM = 13), mostly located on the trunk (n = 36), lower limb (n = 16), upper limb (n = 18), head/neck (n = 18) | NR | OCT features of icicles and dermal ovoid structures with dark borders both significant ($P<.05$) for diagnosis of AHM compared with other study lesions DEJ disruption commonly seen in AHM on OCT (10 of 13 cases) but was also seen in other NMSC, thus, lacked specificity | Limited number of significant OCT features to help identify AHM because OCT only provides architectural, superficial view of a skin lesion but does not offer cellular resolution Weak inter-rater agreement |
| Markowitz et al,[30] 2016, United States | 30 male patients, aged 67–93 y (mean 76 y), all being treated with ingenol mebutate gel 0.015%; 2 patients excluded | 336 lesions (168 clinical AKs, 168 perilesional) | OCT detected 100% (28 of 28) of clinical and 73% (16 of 22) of subclinical lesions at baseline | At day 60, OCT indicated 76% clinical lesion clearance rate (52 of 68) for ingenol mebutate treated areas vs 11% (6 of 55) for untreated areas Clearance rate for subclinical lesions with ingenol mebutate: 88% (21 of 24) vs 43% (6 of 14) | Only 28 subjects, all of whom represented a very similar demographics OCT scans read by single blinded dermatologist |

(continued on next page)

**Table 2**
*(continued)*

| First Author, Year, Country | Population Characteristics | Lesions, Number | Accuracy | Findings/Results | Limitations |
|---|---|---|---|---|---|
| Cheng et al,[8] 2016, Australia | 103 patients (63 M, 40F), aged 31–88 y (median 66 y) | 168 lesions: 52% sBCC, 26% other BCC variants, remainder were AK, SCCIS, other benign inflammatory processes and 2 other malignant tumors<br><br>Lesions located on the trunk (55.4%), upper extremity (18.5%), head/neck (13.7%), lower extremity (12.5%) | sBCC diagnosis Sensitivity 87%, specificity 80%, PPV 83%, NPV 86%<br><br>With high clinical confidence for sBCC (>90%), and high OCT interpreter confidence, an accuracy rate of 89%<br><br>Interobserver agreement: 3 observers of varying experience, κ = 0.596; among 2 experienced observers, κ = 0.766 | Clefting, hyporeflective ovoid structure, and absence of a fully encompassing ovoid structure highly predictive of sBCC<br><br>Good diagnostic accuracy with OCT for diagnosing sBCC and measuring depth in tumors <0.4 mm<br><br>Potential to reduce the need for biopsy in clinically suspected sBCCs with OCT use; careful follow-up required as there is a small risk (5%) of misdiagnosis; a potential 76% biopsy reduction rate of biopsy associated with a 5% error rate<br><br>Good interobserver agreement between experienced and inexperienced observers | Potential pitfall: identified case of amelanotic melanoma that was diagnosed as sBCC clinically and on OCT |
| Meekings et al,[9] 2016 | NR | 40 BCCs (13 nodular, 22 superficial, 5 morpheaform) | NR | Diagnostic criteria for BCC: hyporeflective ovoid structures (40 of 40), dark halo boundaries (38 of 40), epidermal thinning (28 of 40), and collagen compression (14 of 40) | Retrospective study Unblinded interpreters |

| | | | | |
|---|---|---|---|---|
| Olsen et al,[10] 2016, Denmark | 162 patients (90 M, 73 F), mean age 69.4 y | 142 lesions (41 BCCs, 30 AKs, 71 normal skin) located mainly on the head (90 of 142), followed by the trunk (32 of 142) and extremities (20 of 142) | Skilled observers: Diagnosing AK: sensitivity 56%–96%, specificity 52%–83% Diagnosing BCC: sensitivity 86%–95%[a], specificity 81%–98%[a] Diagnosing healthy skin: sensitivity 36%–84%[a], specificity 95%–100% Differentiating NMSC vs healthy skin: sensitivity 94%–100%, specificity 28%–76% Unskilled observers: Diagnosing AK: sensitivity 54%–83%, specificity 52%–65% Diagnosing BCC: sensitivity 66%–85%, specificity 73%–94% Diagnosing healthy skin: sensitivity 20%–52%, specificity 94%–100% Differentiating NMSC vs healthy skin: sensitivity 93%–100%, specificity 21%–54% | Note: skilled observers: 1–10 y of OCT research and 3–28 y clinical experience in dermatology; unskilled observers: no experience in OCT and 1–15 y of clinical experience in dermatology Skilled observers better at interpreting OCT images compared with unskilled observers with a significantly higher sensitivity and specificity in diagnosing BCC and healthy skin; thus, potential increase in diagnostic accuracy with intensified training in OCT For AK: no significant difference in sensitivity or specificity between groups |
| | | | | NMSC lesions overdiagnosed by both groups: resulting in high sensitivity but a mediocre specificity and may be because OCT images of healthy skin were obtained from skin adjacent to NMSC lesions and, thus, may have features of sun damage due to field cancerization Study based on selected good-quality OCT images without significant artifacts from hairs and hyperkeratotic areas: not representative of population |
| Wahrlich et al,[29] 2015, Germany | 130 patients (58 F, 72 M), average age 68.1–61.3 y | 98 BCCs, located on the head, trunk, extremities, 29 other skin diseases | Application of scoring system, Berlin Score Students: sensitivity 92.8%, specificity 24.1% Experts: sensitivity 96.6%, specificity 75.2% | 88% of all diagnoses correctly classified & confirmed by histopathology Invasive SCC most frequent false-positive diagnosis |

(continued on next page)

**Table 2**
*(continued)*

| First Author, Year, Country | Population Characteristics | Lesions, Number | Accuracy | Findings/Results | Limitations |
|---|---|---|---|---|---|
| Maier et al,[12] 2015, Germany | 4 patients (3 F, 1 M) | 14 AK lesions located on the upper extremity undergoing topical ingenol mebutate | NR | OCT features of AK pretreatment: crusts or scaling, epidermal broadening and thickening, ill-defined dermoepidermal boarder, hyperkeratosis During treatment: subepidermal blistering, dermal edema Noninvasive imaging superior to clinical evaluation to detect nonresponding lesions | Case series |
| Ulrich et al,[7] 2015, Germany | 156 patients, aged 33–90 y (median 70 y) | Total: 235 nonpigmented pink lesions suspicious for BCC Histology identified 141 of 235 (60%) as BCCs (44 nBCC, 59 sBCC, 19 sclerosing BCC, 19 other BCC), located mostly on head (41.0%) and upper body (48.8%) | Increase in sensitivity from 90.0% (clinical examination) to 95.7% (clinical + dermoscopy + OCT) (P = .099) Increase in specificity from 28.6% by clinical assessment to 54.3% using dermoscopy and to 75.3% with the addition of OCT (P<.001)[a] PPV: 66.0% (clinical), 75.0% (dermoscopy), 85.2% (OCT) NPV: 65% (clinical), 79.4% (dermoscopy), 92.1% (OCT) | Diagnostic accuracy: increase from 65.8% (clinical) 76.2% (clinical + dermoscopy) to 87.4% (clinical + dermoscopy + OCT) | Caution for rare cases of amelanotic melanoma, which can present as a pink patch, plaque, or nodule |

| Blumetti et al,[13] 2015, Brazil | NR | 39 lesions: 19 melanomas (10 in situ, 9 invasive, with Breslow thickness <1 mm), 15 compound nevi, 5 junctional nevi | NR | Presence of dermal shadows correlated significantly with in situ melanoma (8 in 10 cases, $P = .007$); shadows and loss of bright collagen correlated with invasive melanoma, compared with compound nevi ($P = .002$ and $P<.001$). Hyporeflective band associated with compound nevi (80%) and less frequently found in melanomas (31.5% $P = .007$) Summary: Prescience of dermal shadows and absence of bright collagen most relevant parameters to suggest malignancy Lack of hyporeflective bands on invasive melanomas distinguished this from compound nevi | Small population |

(continued on next page)

**Table 2**
*(continued)*

| First Author, Year, Country | Population Characteristics | Lesions, Number | Accuracy | Findings/Results | Limitations |
|---|---|---|---|---|---|
| Markowitz et al,[6] 2015, United States | 100 patients, >18 y old | 115 clinically challenging BCCs located on the head or neck | Diagnostic accuracy: 57.4% (clinical), 69.6% (dermoscopy), 87.8% (OCT)<br><br>Increase in specificity from 48.9% by clinical assessment to 55.6% using dermoscopy and to 80% with the addition of OCT<br><br>Increase in sensitivity from 62.9% by clinical assessment to 78.6% using dermoscopy and to 92.9% with the addition of OCT<br><br>PPV: 65.7% (clinical), 74.3% (dermoscopy), 87.8% (OCT)<br><br>NPV: 45.8% (clinical), 62.5% (dermoscopy), 87.8% (OCT) | Significant improvement in sensitivity and specificity over clinical or dermoscopic evaluation alone with OCT<br><br>Certainty of diagnosis increased by OCT, with a positive effect on accuracy: increase in accuracy of diagnosis with OCT from 88% to 96% when diagnostic certainty was accounted for | Observational study involving only clinically difficult lesions and, thus, likely underestimates the specificity for obvious lesions |
| Mogensen et al,[37] 2009, Denmark | 104 patients, mean age 69.3 y | 64 BCCs, 1 baso-squamous carcinoma, 39 AKs, 2 malignant melanomas, 9 benign lesions Locations NR | Sensitivity 79%–94%, specificity 85%–96% for all NMSCs depending on experience | | Error rate of 50%–52% with discrimination of AK from BCC, much higher than any other study, likely due to older OCT |
| Gambichler et al,[14] 2007, Germany | 75 patients (42 M, 33 F), aged 15–95 y (mean 54.4) | 92 melanocytic lesions (52 BN, 40 MM), mostly located on the trunk, followed by limbs and head. | NR | OCT of MM: marked architectural disarray and DEJ; large, vertical, icicle-shaped structures | Conventional OCT: not enough clear-cut differences demonstrated between MM and BN to be used |

[a] Indicates statistical significance.

*Abbreviations:* AHM, amelanotic/hypomelanotic melanoma; AK, actinic keratosis; BCC, basal cell carcinoma; BN, benign nevi; DEJ, dermoepidermal junction; F, female; FD-OCT, frequency domain optical coherence tomography; M, male; MM, malignant melanoma; NMSC, nonmelanoma skin cancer; NPV, negative predictive value; NR, not reported; PPV, positive predictive value; sBCC, superficial basal cell carcinoma; SCCIS, squamous cell carcinoma in situ.

these ovoid structures are surrounded by a bright fibrous tumor stroma.[6–11] Additional features described include absence of normal hair follicles and glands as well as prominent dilated vessels in the superficial dermis directed toward the basaloid cell islands.[6–11] Some lesions also have small, well-circumscribed, black/hyporeflective areas inside the tumor nests, representing tumor necrosis (**Fig. 1**).[11]

## Squamous Cell Carcinoma/Actinic Keratosis

Actinic keratosis (AK) is considered to be the initial lesion in a continuum that progresses to invasive squamous cell carcinoma (SCC). While clinically it can be difficult to distinguish between AK and SCC, the distinction is critical in determining appropriate treatment. The use of noninvasive imaging can both improve diagnostic accuracy as well as increase the detection of early subclinical disease states.

On FD-OCT, AKs appear as white streaks in the upper epidermis, indicated by hyperechogenic areas that correspond to hyperkeratotic scale.[10,12] There is thickening of the epidermis with a haphazard pattern in the upper portion, disruption of the normal layered skin architecture as well as ill-defined borders at the DEJ.[10,12] Compared with AKs, SCCs tend to have more epidermal thickening

and haphazard patterning and appear more broadly throughout the FOV (**Figs. 2 and 3**).[10,12]

### Melanoma

Compared with nonmelanoma skin cancer (NMSC), there are only a few studies investigating the use of OCT in pigmented lesions. Studies determined that conventional OCT did not demonstrate enough differences from benign nevi to be used as a diagnostic tool for malignant melanoma (MM).[13,14]

## DYNAMIC OPTICAL COHERENCE TOMOGRAPHY
### Basal Cell Carcinoma

On dermoscopic examination, the finding of arborizing vessels is a key feature in the diagnosis of BCC (**Table 3**). Thus, D-OCT has increased the sensitivity in diagnosing BCCs as it can look at the pattern and distribution of vessels.

On the cross-sectional view, BCCs demonstrate a progressive elongation of perpendicular vessel columns.[15–17]

In the en face view, the blood vessels appear irregular and disorganized, displaying a wide variation in blood vessel caliber.[15–17] In addition, BCCs display a high vessel density both throughout the lesion as well as lining the periphery of the tumor

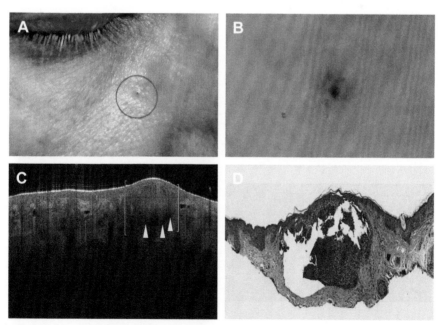

**Fig. 1.** Clinical, dermoscopy, FD-OCT, and histology of a BCC. (*A*) Clinical image of a BCC, appearing as a small pigmented papule (*blue circle*). (*B*) Dermoscopy of a pigmented BCC exhibiting brown/gray ovoid nest surrounded by barbarized vessels. (*C*) Cross-sectional FD-OCT image of a BCC. Features include dark hyporeflective ovoid area (*blue brackets*) with a black rim (*arrowheads*). Note the effaced DEJ above the BCC and the prominent blood vessels in the dermis (*orange arrows*). (*D*) Corresponding histopathology (Haemotoxylin and Eosin).

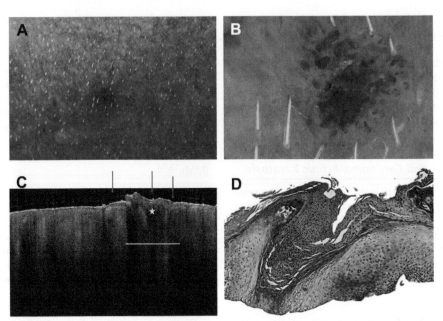

**Fig. 2.** Clinical, dermoscopy, FD-OCT, and histology of an AK. (*A*) Clinical image of an AK appearing as an erythematous, scaly, papule. (*B*) Dermoscopy shows minimal ulceration, some dotted vessels, and a superficial white hyper-reflective scale. (*C*) Cross-sectional FD-OCT image of an AK. Features include localized foci of epidermal thickening (*yellow star*) and hyperkeratotic scale (*orange arrows*). Note the disruption of the DEJ beneath the thickened epidermis. (*D*) Corresponding histopathology (Haemotoxylin and Eosin).

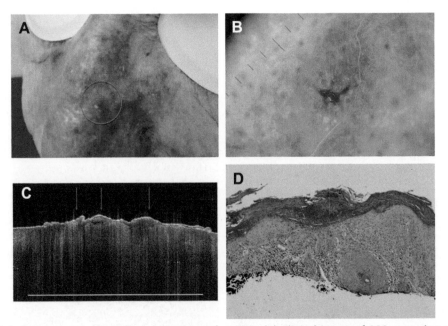

**Fig. 3.** Clinical, dermoscopy, FD-OCT, and histology of an SCC. (*A*) Clinical image of SCC appearing as a small erythematous, scaly papule (*blue circle*). (*B*) Dermoscopy shows ulceration with white hyper-reflective scale. (*C*) Cross-sectional FD-OCT image of an SCC. SCCs appear similar to that of actinic keratosis, although they exhibit more epidermal thickening and hyperkeratotic scale (*orange arrows*). They also appear more broadly throughout the FOV. Note the lack of a distinct DEJ. (*D*) Corresponding histopathology (Haemotoxylin and Eosin).

**Table 3**
Summary of studies investigating the use of optical coherence tomography to evaluate skin cancers: high-definition optical coherence tomography (Skintell)

| First Author, Year, Country | Population Characteristics | Lesions, Number | Accuracy | Findings/Results | Limitations |
|---|---|---|---|---|---|
| Marneffe et al,[24] 2016, Belgium | 36 patients (19 F, 17 M), aged 38–89 y (median 68 y) | 106 lesions (38 AKs, 16 SCCs, 52 normal skin sites), localized mostly on the head/neck region and lower limbs | Experienced user: AK diagnosis: sensitivity 81.6%, specificity 92.6%, PPV 86.1%, NPV 90% SCC diagnosis: sensitivity 93.8%, specificity 98.9%, PPV 93.8%, NPV 98.9% Normal skin diagnosis: sensitivity 92.3%, specificity 88.9%, PPV 88.9%, NPV 92.3% All aforementioned listed numbers: consistently and statistically significantly higher than less-experienced observers | Disrupted DEJ: highly sensitive for invasive SCC, minimizing the false-negative rate Budding/periadnexal collars: enabled ~100% specificity for SCC, minimizing false-positive rate | Hyperkeratotic AKs, thought to be most likely to progress to SCC, excluded from this study because the high refractive index of the keratin interfered with the visualization of the deeper cutaneous layers Results obtained by 3 observers, cannot be extended to all dermatologists Only AKs and SCCs included in the study: did not evaluate discrimination from other diagnosis characterized by dyskeratosis (ie, psoriasis, lichen planus) |

(continued on next page)

**Table 3**
*(continued)*

| First Author, Year, Country | Population Characteristics | Lesions, Number | Accuracy | Findings/Results | Limitations |
|---|---|---|---|---|---|
| Boone et al,[23] 2015, Belgium | 53 patients (25 M, 28 F), age 38–93 y (mean age 65.5 y) | 53 lesions (37 AKs and 16 SCCs), 40 lesions on face, 9 extremities, 4 on the trunk | See Findings/Results | Discriminating SCC from AK and normal skin: Presence of outlined DEJ on cross-sectional imaging suggestive for normal skin or AK vs blurred/not detectable junction suggestive of SCC Sensitivity 100%, specificity 94% Discriminating AK from normal skin: En face mode: atypical honeycomb pattern (sensitivity 100%, specificity 100%); cross-sectional mode: alternating hyperkeratosis/parakeratosis (100% sensitivity, 100% specificity) Discriminating AKs with/without adnexal involvement: En face mode: presence and absence of the cocarde image distinguished AKs with/without adnexal involvement, respectively | Study does not represent a testing set but only a training set Severe hyperkeratotic (>300 μm) lesions excluded due to unclear visualization on HD-OCT; HAK important differential for invasive SCC, so further studies need to be done |

| Boone et al,[18] 2015, Belgium | 50 patients (22 M, 28 F), range from 35 to 87 y (median 66 y) | 50 BCCs: 18 sBCC, 19 nBCC, and 13 iBCC, located mainly on the trunk (62%), followed by head/neck (26%) and limbs (12%) 50 non-BCC (25 AKs, 12 melanocytic lesions, 10 sebaceous hyperplasias, 3 hemangiomas) | NR | Gray to dark lobulated structures present in 48 of 50 (96%) BCCs, in none of the AKs, and in all other BCC imitators; lobular structures characterized by a cockade feature (bright outer rim) in 37 of 50 (74%) BCCs and also present in 6 of 10 (60%) of sebaceous hyperplasias, but absent in other BCC imitators<br>sBCC: lobular structures connected to the epidermis (swallow nests), type A vessels (short fine holes), absence of stretched fibers<br>nBCC: lobular structures, stretched fibers, type B vessel (small branched holes)<br>iBCC: lobular structures, stretched fibers, type C vessels (large branched holes) |
| Gambichler et al,[25] 2015, Germany | 64 patients | Total 93 melanocytic lesions: 66 BN (23 compound nevi, 20 JN, 10 dermal nevi, 9 DN, 2 nevoid lentigo, 2 blue nevi) and 27 melanomas (23 superficial spreading, 2 LMM, 1 nodular, 1 acral lentiginous melanoma) | HD-OCT for MM: sensitivity 74.1%, specificity 92.4%, PPV 80%, NPV 89.7% | HD-OCT risk parameters for MM: large roundish pagetoid cells, atypical cell clusters in DEJ, totally disarranged epidermal/dermal pattern, bright bizarre dermal horizontal streaks, large vertical icicle-shaped structures<br>HD-OCT has moderate diagnostic potential in differentiating benign vs malignant MSL, however, is inferior to RCM | High false-negative rates in very thin melanomas and high false positive rates in dysplastic nevi<br>Small sample size<br>Only one blinded observer<br>Used preliminary micromorphologic HD-OCT features of MSL |

(continued on next page)

**Table 3**
*(continued)*

| First Author, Year, Country | Population Characteristics | Lesions, Number | Accuracy | Findings/Results | Limitations |
|---|---|---|---|---|---|
| Boone et al,[26] 2014, Belgium | 26 patients | 26 melanocytic lesions (3 JN, 8 compound nevi, 1 DN, 1 blue nevus, 9 dysplastic nevi, 4 melanoma) | NR | HD-OCT melanoma: Cross-sectional mode: atypical large melanocytes in the upper part of the acanthotic epidermis, altered DEJ with irregular and broadened rete ridges, atypical cells tended to for junctional sheets or irregular junctional aggregates distorting the rete ridges En face mode: cobblestone or irregular honeycomb pattern in superficial layer, epidermal disarray in areas of pagetoid spread, atypical melanocytes in the upper part of dermis | Pilot study, small number of lesions |
| Gambichler et al,[27] 2014, Germany | n = 48 | NR | NR | Showed that pagetoid cells, fusion of rete ridges, and junctional and/or dermal nests with atypical cells significantly more frequently seen in melanoma when compared with benign nevi Because of higher resolution: HD-OCT has higher diagnostic potential in differentiating between benign and malignant melanocytic lesions compared with conventional OCT | Absence of suspicious HD-OCT features in some thin melanomas is a major limitation of HD-OCT |

| Study | Patients | Lesions | Sensitivity/Specificity | Findings | Comments |
|---|---|---|---|---|---|
| Li et al,[19] 2014, Germany | 43 patients (25 M, 18 F), aged 38–87 y (mean 65.3 y) | 43 total lesions: 22 BCC, 10 fibrous papules of the face, 5 AK, 3 intradermal nevi, 2 SCC, 1 sebaceous hyperplasia | Experienced investigator diagnosing BCC: sensitivity of 86.4%, specificity of 90.5% Inexperienced investigator diagnosing BCC: sensitivity 77.3%, specificity 81% | Good interobserver agreement between experienced and inexperienced investigators (concordance of 77% and 81%, respectively) | |
| Gambichler et al,[20] 2014, Germany | 20 patients (15 M, 5 F), mean age 67.1 y | 25 BCCs (13 solid type, 9 superficial type, 3 infiltrative type) | NR | En face mode: lobulated nodules were seen in 21 of 25 lesions (84%, $P = .0014$), peripheral rimming in 18 of 25 (72%, $P = .046$), epidermal disarray 18 of 25 (72%, $P = .046$) and variably refractile stroma in 22 BCCs (88%, $P = .0003$) Cross-section: destruction of layering in 19 of 25 BCCs (76%, $P = .0164$) | Unable to differentiate different BCC subtypes |
| Maier et al,[21] 2013, Germany | 14 M patients, aged 51–82 y | 22 BCCs (11 nodular, 5 superficial, 4 infiltrative, 1 pigmented, 1 adenoid) | NR | En face mode: lobulated nodules (20 of 22), peripheral rimming (17 of 22), epidermal disarray (21 of 22), dilated vessels (11 of 22), and variably refractile stromal (19 of 22) Slice mode: gray/dark oval structures (18 of 22), peripheral rimming (13 of 22), destruction of layering (22 of 22), dilated vessels (7 of 22), peritumoral bright stroma (11 of 22) | |

*Abbreviations:* BN, benign nevi; DN, dysplastic nevi; F, female; HAK, hypertrophic actinic keratosis; iBCC, invasive BCC; JN, junctional nevi; LMM, lentigo maligna melanoma; M, male; MSL, melanocytic skin lesions; nBCC, nodular BCC; NPV, negative predictive value; PPV, positive predictive value; sBCC, superficial BCC; SES, skin entrance signal.

islands, demarcating the tumor from normal skin (**Figs. 4 and 5**).[15–17]

### Squamous Cell Carcinoma/Actinic Keratosis

On the en face view, AKs generally appear as a reticular network of vessels similar to normal skin, although tend to be slightly broader and more irregular.[15] In contrast, SCCs appear significantly different as regularly distributed dotted structures immediately below the epidermis (**Figs. 6 and 7**).[15]

### Malignant Melanoma

Examining the vasculature of melanocytic lesions with D-OCT in the en face view has been shown to be useful in differentiating benign from malignant lesions. Congenital nevi usually display a pattern of regularly distributed dotted structures immediately below the epidermis, with a pattern usually comparable with surrounding skin.[15] In contrast, melanoma shows densely clustered red dots in the superficial dermis that present a chaotic and irregular vascular distribution compared with nevi.[15] As tumor thickness increases, the red dots aggregate to long linear vessels with angulated branches and irregular size (**Fig. 8**).[15–17]

## HIGH-DEFINITION OPTICAL COHERENCE TOMOGRAPHY
### Basal Cell Carcinoma

HD-OCT has improved cellular resolution compared with conventional FD-OCT and has been shown to not only correctly identify BCCs

from its clinical imitators but also distinguish between different BCC subtypes (**Table 4**).

On en face mode, BCCs exhibit lobulated nodules, peripheral rimming, epidermal disarray, and variably refractile stroma.[18–21] On cross-sectional mode, BCCs have destruction of layering.[18–21]

Boone and colleagues[18] determined that the appearance of gray to dark lobulated structures with a bright outer rim (cockade feature), on both en face and cross-sectional imaging modes, were present in almost all BCCs and are, thus, considered the hallmark for diagnosis.[18] These lobular structures were absent in all AKs; although present in other BCC imitators, only sebaceous hyperplasias were found to also have a bright outer rim.[18] When the lobular structures were connected with a hair follicle, this was found to be pathognomonic of sebaceous hyperplasia and is one way to differentiate them from BCC.[18] All BCCs had increased vascularization within the superficial papillary dermis, displayed as holes on HD-OCT, although the appearance differed between subtype.

BCC subtype could be classified based on the type of lobular structures, the presence or absence of stretched fibers in the stroma (stretching effect), and the dominant vascular pattern present.[18]

Superficial BCCs (sBCCs) were the only BCC subtype to have lobular structures directly connected to the epidermis (swallow nests), type A vessels (short, fine holes), and the absence of stretched fibers (**Figs. 9 and 10**).[18] In contrast, nodular BCCs (nBCCs) and invasive BCCs (iBCCs) had lobular structures with cockade not connected to the epidermis and almost all of them

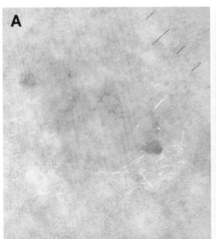 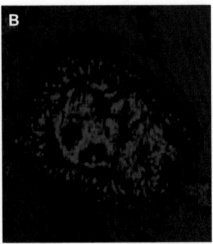

**Fig. 4.** Dermoscopy and en face view of BCC on D-OCT: (*A*) Dermoscopy of BCC with pink-white shiny background, focal ulceration, arborizing vessels. (*B*) En face D-OCT of BCC shows disarray of thin, irregular vessels that are variable in size compared with the normal facial vessels. In comparison with more aggressive tumors, such as melanoma, the vascular pattern appears confined to the tumor.

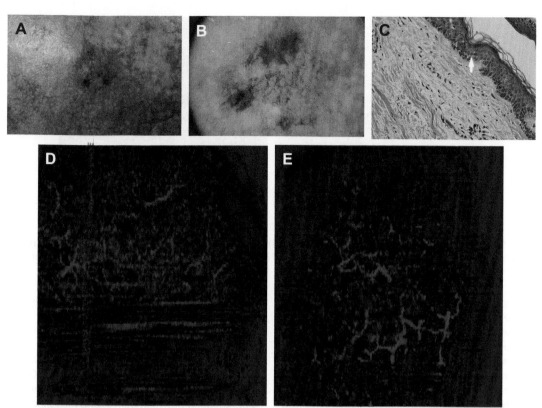

**Fig. 5.** Clinical, dermoscopy, histology an MM in situ on the forehead (*A–C*). En face D-OCT of a benign nevus (*D*) and a melanoma in situ (*E*). (*A*) Clinical image of melanoma in situ on the forehead, presented as a large, asymmetric pigmented lesion. (*B*) Dermoscopy shows asymmetric pigmented follicular opening, and slate gray dots and globules. (*C*) Corresponding histopathology (Haemotoxylin and Eosin). Arrow is pointing to the atypical melanocytes in the dermal-epidermal junction. (*D*) Benign nevi show regularly distributed vessels, comparable with the surrounding normal skin. (*E*) Melanoma in situ exhibit long linear vessels that appear broken and irregular and have a chaotic distribution.

had a stretching effect (see **Figs. 9** and **10**).[18] BCC subtypes can be differentiated by the vascular patterns that they display, as nBCCs are characterized by small, branched vessels, whereas iBCCs exhibit large, branched holes.[18]

## Squamous Cell Carcinoma/Actinic Keratosis

On cross-sectional (vertical) sections, most AKs displayed a clear DEJ outline. In contrast, SCCs displayed irregular reflective buddings projecting from the epidermis deep into the dermis,

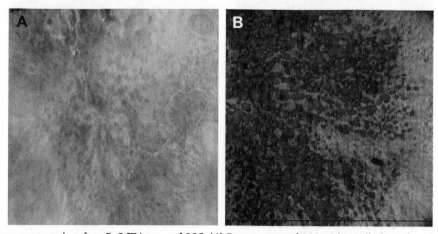

**Fig. 6.** Dermoscopy and en face D-OCT image of SCC. (*A*) Dermoscopy of SCC with small, dotted, and glomerular vessels distributed in packed clusters. (*B*) En-face D-OCT of SCC shows that vessels appear dotted in morphology.

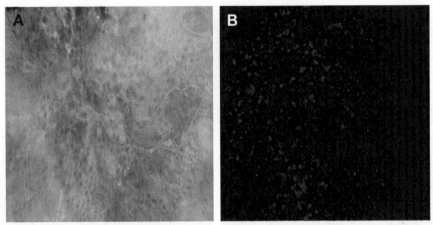

**Fig. 7.** Dermoscopy and en face D-OCT image of SCC. (*A*) Dermoscopy of SCC with small, dotted, and glomerular vessels distributed in packed clusters. (*B*) En-face D-OCT of SCC shows that vessels appear dotted in morphology similar to what is seen on dermoscopy.

interrupting or obscuring the DEJ.[22–24] All SCCs and AKs had alternating hyperkeratosis and parakeratosis as well as alternating atrophy and hypertrophy.[22–24]

On en face HD-OCT, the extent of disruption of the honeycomb pattern in the epidermis was found to correlate with the severity of AK and the diagnosis of SCC. A mildly atypical honeycomb pattern was displayed in most AKs, whereas a severely atypical honeycomb pattern was seen in 100% of SCCs.[22–24] In addition, about 50% of AKs and all SCCs had adnexal involvement, where the classic *cocarde* image (perifollicular hyporeflective band surrounded by a thin dark ring) was replaced by atypical keratinocytes cuffing the hair follicle.[22–24] This finding is significant as studies have shown that AKs with follicular extension have an increased risk of developing into SCCs (**Figs. 11** and **12**).[23]

## Malignant Melanoma

Because of higher cellular resolution, HD-OCT has been found to have a higher diagnostic potential in differentiating between benign and malignant melanocytic lesions compared with FD-OCT.

Cellular findings of MM on cross-sectional HD-OCT include atypical large roundish pagetoid cells, junctional and/or dermal nests with atypical cell clusters, altered DEJ, and irregular and broadened rete ridges.[25–27]

Findings on en face mode include the following: superficial layer showed cobblestone or irregular honeycomb pattern; epidermal disarray observed

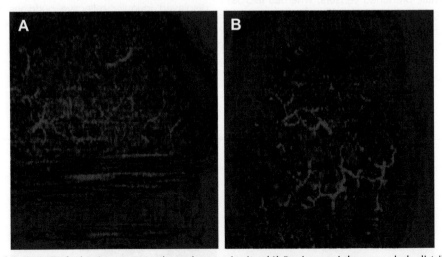

**Fig. 8.** En face D-OCT of a benign nevus and a melanoma in situ. (*A*) Benign nevi show regularly distributed vessels similar to the surrounding normal skin. (*B*) Melanomas in situ exhibit long linear vessels that appear broken and irregular and have a chaotic distribution that comprises the entire en face FOV.

**Table 4**
Summary of studies investigating the use of optical coherence tomography to evaluate skin cancers: dynamic optical coherence tomography/speckle-variance optical coherence tomography

| First Author, Year, Country | Population Characteristics | Lesions, Number | Accuracy | Findings/Results | Limitations |
|---|---|---|---|---|---|
| Ulrich et al,[15] 2016, Germany | NR | NR | NR | Superficial BCC: cross-sectional view: progressive elongation of perpendicular vessel columns; en face view: variation in the calibers of the blood vessels, disorganized with a multitude of minute vessels<br>AK: D-OCT: reticular network on en face view, which resembles the network of normal skin but vessels form a larger caliber and a slightly irregular, broader network<br>Bowens/SCCIS: enface view: vessels appear dotted or semicircular<br>Melanoma: densely clustered red dots may be visible in the superficial dermis; red dots aggregate to linear structures with increase in tumor thickness | NR |
| Markowitz et al,[16] 2016, United States | NR | 4 lesions (sebaceous hyperplasia, BCC, MM in situ, pigmented AK) | NR | En face:<br>BCC: had a focal vascular pattern with an erratic vascular organization compared with benign sebaceous tumor<br>Normal telangiectasia with minimal focal vascular irregularity with pigmented AK<br>MMIS: revealed diffuse thin irregular vessels dispersed throughout the entire field | Case series |
| De Carvalho et al,[17] 2016, Italy | NR | 1 | NR | Benign lentiginous:<br>Cross-section: thin regular columns on transversal section, and regularly distributed dots or short curved lines, progressively assuming a regular reticulated architecture with depth in en face view; did not differ from the vascular pattern of normal surrounding skin<br>Melanoma:<br>Cross-sectional: vessels organized in larger vertical columns, irregularly distributed<br>En face: vascular pattern characterized by numerous densely packed dots progressively becoming irregular cloudlike structures with depth<br>CD31 staining confirmed the correspondence of SV-OCT images | 1 patient |

*Abbreviations:* NR, not reported; SCCIS, SCC in situ.

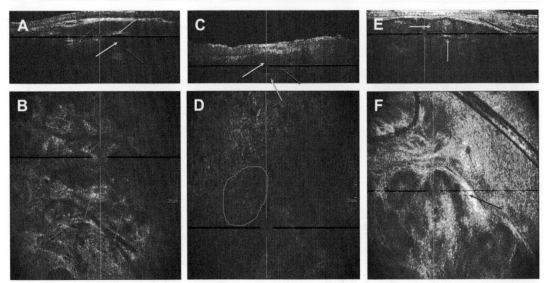

**Fig. 9.** HD-OCT features of infiltrative, sBCC, and nodular BCC. (*A, B*) Infiltrative BCC. Elongated, gray to black lobular structures can be observed, separated with deeper dermal localization and more pronounced stretching effect (*pink arrow*). The typical cockade image is present: the gray core (*yellow arrow*) of the lobular structure surrounded by the dark inner layer (*red arrow*) and bright peripheral outer rim (*green arrow*). There is an abundant of large, dilated branched vessels observed (*dark green arrow*). (*C, D*) sBCC. A hemispherical nestlike, dark-gray structure connected to the epidermis on cross-sectional images. Notice the increased and altered microvasculature (*dark green encircled area*). (*E, F*) Nodular BCC. Intradermal gray to dark colored structures with typical cockade feature present: a gray core (*yellow arrow*), an inner dark rim (*red arrow*), and an outer peripheral bright rim (*light green arrow*). These lobules cause abnormal dermal architecture in both cross-sectional and en face images. There is a stretching effect of the tumor on the fibrous structures, appearing as variably reflective stroma, located between lobular structures (*pink arrow*). (*Courtesy of* Mark Boone, MD, Lennik, Belgium.)

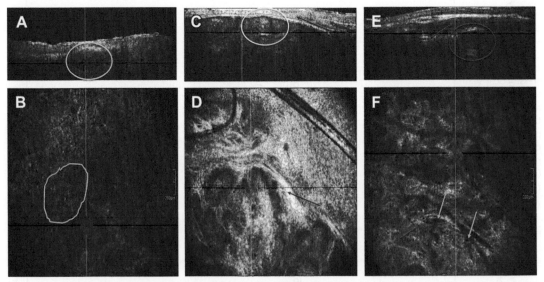

**Fig. 10.** HD-OCT features of sBCC, nodular, and infiltrative BCC. (*A, B*) sBCC. A hemispherical nestlike, dark-gray structure connected to the epidermis on cross-sectional images (*blue circle*). Notice the increased and altered microvasculature (*green encircled area*). (*C, D*) Nodular BCC. Intradermal gray to dark colored structures with typical cockade feature present: a gray core, an inner dark rim, and an outer peripheral bright rim (*yellow circle*). These lobules cause abnormal dermal architecture in both cross-sectional and en face images. There is a stretching effect of the tumor on the fibrous structures, appearing as variably reflective stroma, located between lobular structures (*pink arrow*). (*E, F*) Infiltrative BCC. Elongated, gray to black lobular structures can be observed, separated with deeper dermal localization and more pronounced stretching effect (*pink arrow*). The typical cockade image is present (*red circle*): the gray core of the lobular structure surrounded by the dark inner layer and bright peripheral outer rim. There is an abundant of large, dilated, branched vessels observed (*green arrows*). (*Courtesy of* Mark Boone, MD, Lennik, Belgium.)

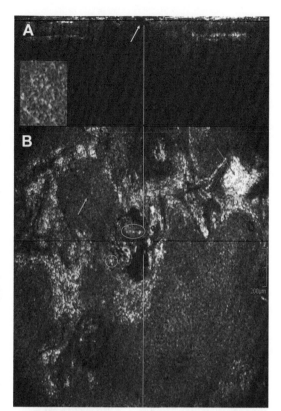

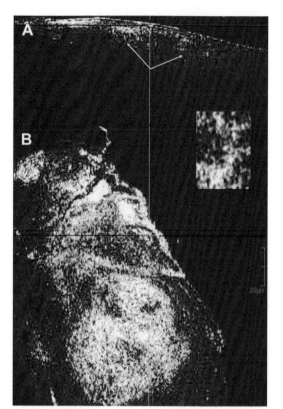

**Fig. 11.** Non-Bowenoid AK with adnexal involvement. Cross-sectional and en face HD-OCT image of AK with adnexal involvement. (*A*) In the cross-sectional mode, a follicular structure (*yellow arrow*) interrupts the subepidermal dark band. (*B*) In the en face view, you can see repression of normal adnexal epithelium by atypical cells, leading to the disa - ppearance of the classic cocarde image, which is replaced by atypical keratinocytes cuffing the hair follicle (hair follicle, *green arrow*; atypical cells, *green circle*). The borders of keratinocytes comprising the mildly atypical honeycomb pattern are more irregular and brighter and contours of nuclei are more masked (*close-up*). Notice the alternating hyperkeratosis (*red arrow*) with parakeratosis (*brown arrow*) that can be seen in both views. (*Courtesy of* Mark Boone, MD, Lennik, Belgium.)

**Fig. 12.** Cross-sectional and en face HD-OCT image of SCC. (*A*) Cross-sectional HD-OCT image of an SCC. Notice the irregular budding of epidermis deeper into the dermis, obscuring the DEJ (*yellow arrows*). (*B*) En face HD-OCT of an SCC shows severe architectural disarray of the epidermis and dermis. Severely atypical honeycomb pattern (*close-up*). The DEJ is no longer present. Acantholysis is pronounced. (*Courtesy of* Mark Boone, MD, Lennik, Belgium.)

in areas of pagetoid spread; atypical melanocytes observed in the upper part of dermis (**Figs. 13 and 14**).[25–27]

## LIMITATIONS

Two cases of amelanotic melanomas being misdiagnosed as BCCs on FD-OCT have been reported.[7,8,28] Clinicians must remain cautious about using this modality to assist noninvasive diagnosis of clinically uncertain amelanotic or hypomelanotic skin lesions because some OCT features are nonspecific and overlap with

amelanotic melanomas.[7,8,28] Further studies need to be done to see if D-OCT can help to differentiate this.

Olsen and colleagues[10] and Wahrlich and colleagues[29] used FD-OCT to show that both experts and nonexperts overdiagnosed NMSC lesions resulting in a high sensitivity but only an average specificity. This finding is thought to be because the OCT images of healthy skin were obtained from skin next to NMSC lesions and, therefore, likely had features of sun damage due to field cancerization.[10,29]

Gambichler and colleagues[27] demonstrated a limitation for HD-OCT in melanoma diagnosis in that accuracy depends on tumor thickness and the presence of borderline lesions. In their study, this is indicated by a high false-negative rate in very thin melanomas and a high false-positive rate in dysplastic nevi, making it still inferior to RCM.[27]

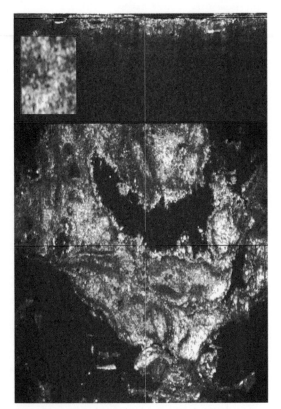

**Fig. 13.** Bowenoid AK. Cross-sectional (slice) and en face HD-OCT images. This lesion represents a carcinoma in situ with full- thickness atypia involving the epidermis and adnexal structures. A complete disarranged epidermal pattern and acantholysis are observed. (*Courtesy of* Mark Boone, MD, Lennik, Belgium.)

All noninvasive imaging devices were limited as a result of increased lesion thickness; therefore, clinically apparent lesions, such as hypertrophic AKs, lead to difficulty in visualizing the deeper structures.[23,24] This difficulty was even an issue with FD-OCT, despite its increased depth.

## MONITORING OF SURGICAL AND NONSURGICAL SKIN CANCER THERAPIES

With the advent of new nonsurgical therapeutic options for NMSC, such as topical chemotherapy, immunomodulators, and photodynamic therapy, noninvasive imaging is useful in the monitoring of treatment progress as well as determining treatment efficacy.[30–33] Noninvasive treatment monitoring is also useful in patients with lesions on cosmetically sensitive areas of the face, as these patients often refuse posttreatment biopsy confirmation.

An additional use specific to all OCT devices is defining tumor margins before surgery. Studies have shown that the OCT margin was always on

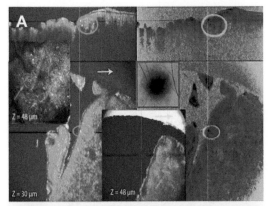

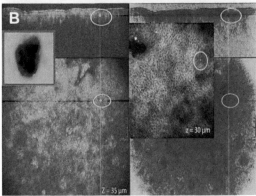

**Fig. 14.** Pagetoid melanoma. (*A, B*) Pagetoid melanocytosis is represented by the presence of large melanocytes (twice the size of neighboring keratinocyte) with abundant reflective cytoplasm (*green circle*) and sometimes characterized by a prominent hyporeflective nucleus depending on the image focus (*white circle*). (*A*) The pagetoid cells may be more elongated with variable morphology of the branches. Thick branches can be observed by HD-OCT (*green arrow*). Thin, bright filamentous structures are only observed by RCM (*blue arrow*). On the HD-OCT en face images, the 2-mm diameter plastic ring can be observed (*yellow arrow*). (*Courtesy of* Mark Boone, MD, Lennik, Belgium.)

or within the clinical defect boundary.[34–37] Delineating tumor margins preoperatively can potentially reduce the number of stages required.[34–37]

## SUMMARY

OCT is a noninvasive imaging technique that produces highly sensitive and specific images of tissue microstructure. This ability allows for improved diagnostic accuracy for a variety of both benign and malignant skin conditions. FD-OCT, D-OCT, and HD-OCT are the main devices reviewed in this article; all have been shown to be useful for NMSCs and precancerous growths. More research is currently being done to understand the role of these devices with pigmented lesions in differentiating melanoma. Other unique benefits of OCT given its depth and broader FOV are both monitoring lesion treatment undergoing nonsurgical therapy and in delineating margins before surgery.

## ACKNOWLEDGEMENTS

The authors would like to thank Marc Boone, MD for contributing the HD-OCT images.

## REFERENCES

1. Schwartz M, Siegel D, Markowitz O. Commentary on the diagnostic utility of non-invasive imaging devices for field cancerization. Exp Dermatol 2016; 25:855–6.

2. Schmitz L, Reinhold U, Bierhoff E, et al. Optical coherence tomography: its role in daily dermatological practice. J Dtsch Dermatol Ges 2013; 11(6):499–507.

3. Gambichler T, Jaedicke V, Terras S. Optical coherence tomography in dermatology: technical and clinical aspects. Arch Dermatol Res 2011;303:457–73.

4. Gambichler T, Pljaki A, Schmitz L. Recent advances in clinical application of optical coherence tomography of human skin. Clin Cosmet Investig Dermatol 2015;8:345–54.

5. Jemef GB, Gniadecka M, Ulrich J. Ultrasound in dermatology. Part I. High frequency ultrasound. Eur J Dermatol 2000;10:492–7.

6. Markowitz O, Schwartz M, Feldman E, et al. Evaluation of optical coherence tomography as a means of identifying earlier stage basal cell carcinomas while reducing the use of diagnostic biopsy. J Clin Aesthet Dermatol 2015;8(10):14–20.

7. Ulrich M, von Braunmuehl T, Kurzen H, et al. The sensitivity and specificity of optical coherence tomography for the assisted diagnosis of non-pigmented basal cell carcinoma: an observational study. Br J Dermatol 2015;173(2):428–35. Available at: https://www.ncbi.nlm.nih.gov/PubMed/25904111.

8. Cheng HM, Lo S, Scolyer R, et al. Accuracy of optical coherence tomography for the diagnosis of superficial basal cell carcinoma: a prospective, consecutive, cohort study of 168 cases. Br J Dermatol 2016;175(6):1290–300.

9. Meekings A, Utz S, Ulrich M, et al. Differentiation of basal cell carcinoma subtypes in multi-beam swept source optical coherence tomography (MSS-OCT). J Drugs Dermatol 2016;15(5):545–50.

10. Olsen J, Themstrup L, De Carvalho N, et al. Diagnostic accuracy of optical coherence tomography in actinic keratosis and basal cell carcinoma. Photodiagnosis Photodyn Ther 2016;16:44–9.

11. Hussain A, Themstrup L, Jemec GBE. Optical coherence tomography in the diagnosis of basal cell carcinoma. Arch Dermatol Res 2015;307:1–10.

12. Maier T, Cekovic D, Ruzicka T, et al. Treatment monitoring of topical ingenol mebutate in actinic keratoses with the combination of optical coherence tomography and reflectance confocal microscopy: a case series. Br J Dermatol 2015;172(3):816–8.

13. Blumetti T, Cohen M, Gomes E, et al. Optical coherence tomography (OCT) features of nevi and melanomas and their association with intraepidermal or dermal involvement: a pilot study. J Am Acad Dermatol 2015;73(2):315–7.

14. Gambichler T, Regeniter P, Bechara F, et al. Characterization of benign and malignant melanocytic skin lesions using optical coherence tomography in vivo. J Am Acad Dermatol 2007;57(4):629–37.

15. Ulrich M, Themstrup L, de Carvalho N, et al. Dynamic optical coherence tomography in dermatology. Dermatology 2016;232:298–311.

16. Markowitz O, Schwartz M, Minhas S, et al. Speckle-variance optical coherence tomography: a novel approach to skin cancer characterization using vascular patterns. Dermatol Online J 2016;22(4) [pii:13030/qt7w10290r].

17. De Carvalho N, Ciardo S, Cesinaro AM, et al. In vivo micro-angiography by means of speckle-variance optical coherence tomography (SV-OCT) is able to detect microscopic vascular changes in nevus to melanoma transition. J Eur Acad Dermatol Venereol 2015;30:e29–108.

18. Boone M, Suppa M, Pellacani G, et al. High-definition optical coherence tomography algorithm for discrimination of basal cell carcinoma from clinical BCC imitators and differentiation between common subtypes. J Eur Acad Dermatol Venereol 2015;29: 1771–80.

19. Li G, Tietze JK, Tao X, et al. High-definition optical coherence tomography in the diagnosis of basal cell carcinoma evaluated by an experienced versus inexperienced investigator. Clin Exp Dermatol Res 2014;5:4.

20. Gambichler T, Plura I, Kampilafkos P, et al. Histopathological correlates of basal cell carcinoma in the slice and en face imaging modes of high-definition optical coherence tomography. Br J Dermatol 2014;170:1358–61.

21. Maier T, Braun-Falco M, Hintz T, et al. Morphology of basal cell carcinoma in high definition optical coherence tomography: en-face and slice imaging mode, and comparison with histology. J Eur Acad Dermatol Venereol 2013;27(1):e97–104.

22. Malvehy J. A new vision of actinic keratosis beyond visible clinical lesions. J Eur Acad Dermatol Venereol 2015;29(1):3–8.

23. Boone MA, Marneffe A, Suppa M, et al. High-definition optical coherence tomography algorithm for the discrimination of actinic keratosis from normal skin and from squamous cell carcinoma. J Eur Acad Dermatol Venereol 2015;29:1606–15.

24. Marneffe A, Suppa M, Miyamoto M, et al. Validation of a diagnostic algorithm for the discrimination of actinic keratosis from normal skin and squamous cell carcinoma by means of high-definition optical coherence tomography. Exp Dermatol 2016;25:684–7.

25. Gambichler T, Schmid-Wendtner MH, Plura I, et al. A multicenter pilot study investigating high-definition optical coherence tomography in the differentiation of cutaneous melanoma and melanocytic nevi. J Eur Acad Dermatol Venereol 2015;29(3):537–41.

26. Boone M, Norrenberg S, Jemec G, et al. High-definition optical coherence tomography imaging of melanocytic lesions: a pilot study. Arch Dermatol Res 2014;306:11–26.

27. Gambichler T, Plura I, Schmid-Wendtner MH, et al. High-definition optical coherence tomography of melanocytic skin lesions. J Biophotonics 2014;8(8):681–6.

28. Maher NG, Blumetti TP, Gomes EE, et al. Melanoma diagnosis may be a pitfall for optical coherence tomography assessment of equivocal amelanotic or hypomelanotic skin lesions. Br J Dermatol 2016. [Epub ahead of print].

29. Wahrlich C, Alawi SA, Batz S, et al. Assessment of a scoring system for basal cell carcinoma with multi-beam optical coherence tomography. J Eur Acad Dermatol Venereol 2015;29:1562–9.

30. Markowitz O, Schwartz M, Feldman E, et al. Defining field cancerization of the skin using noninvasive optical coherence tomography imaging to detect and monitor actinic keratosis in ingenol mebutate 0.015%-treated patients. J Clin Aesthet Dermatol 2016;9(5):18–25.

31. Banzhaf C, Themstrup L, Ring H, et al. Optical coherence tomography imaging of non-melanoma skin cancer undergoing imiquimod therapy. Skin Res Technol 2014;20:170–6.

32. Themstrup L, Banzhaf CA, Mogensen M, et al. Optical coherence tomography imaging of non-melanoma skin cancer undergoing photodynamic therapy reveals subclinical residual lesions. Photodiagnosis Photodyn Ther 2014;11:7–12.

33. Hussain AA, Themstrup L, Nurnberg BM, et al. Adjunct use of optical coherence tomography increases the detection of recurrent basal cell carcinoma over clinical and dermoscopic examination alone. Photodiagnosis Photodyn Ther 2016;14:178–84.

34. Alawi SA, Kuck M, Wahrlich C, et al. Optical coherence tomography for presurgical margin assessment of non-melanoma skin cancer- a practical approach. Exp Dermatol 2013;22:547–51.

35. Wang KX, Meekings A, Fluhr JW, et al. Optical coherence tomography-based optimization of Mohs micrographic surgery of basal cell carcinoma: a pilot study. Dermatol Surg 2013;39:627–33.

36. Coleman AJ, Penney GP, Richardson TJ, et al. Automated registration of optical coherence tomography and dermoscopy in the assessment of sub-clinical spread in basal cell carcinoma. Comput Aided Surg 2014;19:1–12.

37. Mogensen M, Joergensen TM, Nürnberg BM, et al. Assessment of optical coherence tomography imaging in the diagnosis of non- melanoma skin cancer and benign lesions versus normal skin: observer-blinded evaluation by dermatologists and pathologists. Dermatol Surg 2009;35:965–72.

# Electrical Impedance Spectroscopy in Skin Cancer Diagnosis

Ralph P. Braun, MD[a],*, Johanna Mangana, MD[a],
Simone Goldinger, MD[a], Lars French, MD[a],
Reinhard Dummer, MD[a], Ashfaq A. Marghoob, MD[b]

## KEYWORDS

- Melanoma • Basal cell carcinoma • Skin cancer • Squamous cell carcinoma • Nevus
- Electrical impedance • Diagnosis

## KEY POINTS

- Electrical impedance spectroscopy (EIS) is a noninvasive method of diagnosing skin cancer based on differences in electrical impendence between normal and abnormal skin.
- EIS is best performed by physicians who are trained to clinically detect seborrheic keratoses because these lesions are frequently inaccurately classified as malignant by EIS.
- EIS is safe with a high sensitivity in melanoma detection for lesions that are deemed suspicious on clinical and dermoscopic examination.

## INTRODUCTION

Electrical impedance spectroscopy (EIS) is a noninvasive method that aims to help diagnose skin cancer. It is based on measuring electrical impedance in normal (banal) and abnormal (skin cancer) skin and using these measurements to differentiate nevi from melanoma.[1] EIS has been studied since the 1980s and the technique available is now commercially in some countries. Normal and abnormal tissues differ with respect to cell size, shape, orientation, compactness, and structure of cell membranes. These different properties on a cellular level influence the ability of the cells to conduct and store electricity, which is reflected in differences in EIS measurements.

## TECHNOLOGICAL EQUIPMENT

The EIS device consists of a handheld probe equipped with a disposable electrode that is applied directly on the skin (Fig. 1). This probe is connected to a small electrical device that is connected to a touch screen monitor via a cable (Fig. 2). The latest generation of the EIS device permits integration of dermoscopy images into the patient chart together with the EIS measurements data. This feature permits the clinician to integrate the clinical, dermoscopic, and EIS information to augment the cognition of the operator in his or her decision making.

### Electrode

The "microinvasive" electrode of the EIS machine only penetrates to the depth of the stratum corneum (Fig. 3). The surface of each electrode is furnished with small gold covered microinvasive pins. These pins have a triangular shape and approximately 150 μm high with a 170-μm triangular base. These spicules penetrate into the stratum corneum and have a sand paperlike feel; the application of the electrode is painless. The electrode can obtain several measurements and can be

---

[a] Department of Dermatology, University Hospital Zürich, Gloriastr 31, 8091 Zürich, Switzerland; [b] Dermatology Service, Department of Medicine, Memorial Sloan Kettering Cancer Center, 275 York Avenue, New York, NY 10065, USA
* Corresponding author. Department of Dermatology, University Hospital Zurich, Gloriastr 31, Zurich 8091 CHE, Switzerland.
*E-mail address:* Ralph.Braun@usz.ch

Dermatol Clin 35 (2017) 489–493
http://dx.doi.org/10.1016/j.det.2017.06.009
0733-8635/17/© 2017 Elsevier Inc. All rights reserved.

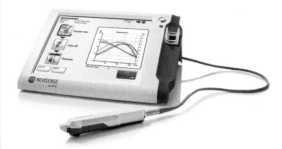

Fig. 1. Nevisense device including hand piece and touch screen monitor. (*Courtesy of* SciBase, Stockholm, Sweden; with permission.)

used on multiple lesions per patient. Because the electrode does penetrate the stratum corneum, it must be discarded after each patient.

## Frequencies

The EIS system measures bioimpedance of the skin at 35 different frequencies, logarithmically distributed between 1.0 and 2.5 MHz, at 4 different depths using 10 permutations. The depth selectivity is measured by using different bars of electrodes (**Fig. 4**). The spatial localization of the sense pin and depth pin determines the 4 depths of penetration calculations used in EIS measurements. In general, impedance at low frequencies is related to the resistive properties of the extracellular environment and impedance at high frequencies is related to the resistive properties of the intracellular and extracellular environment and the capacitive properties (reactance) of the cell membranes. The applied voltage and resulting

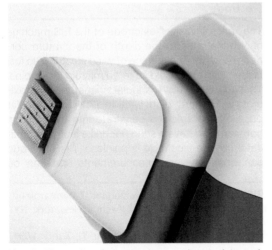

Fig. 2. Electrode of the Nevisense electrical impedance spectroscopy device. (*Courtesy of* SciBase, Stockholm, Sweden; with permission.)

current is limited to 150 mV and 75 µA, respectively. The electrical current cannot be perceived by the patient and a complete electrical impedance measurement study takes less than 10 seconds to perform.

## Measurements

The measurement outcome of an EIS measurement is magnitude and phase shift at each frequency included in the spectrum. The measurements are displayed as curves of magnitude and phase shift at 4 different depths (different colors), and 10 permutations at various frequencies (x axis). Before the application of the electrode and before any measurements are taken, the skin site of interest be moistened with 0.9% saline solution for at least 30 seconds. For each lesion being investigated, the EIS measurements must be performed twice. The first measurement is called the reference measurement and this is obtained on healthy "normal" skin located at least 2 to 3 cm away from the lesion of interest. This reference measurement can even be obtained on the contralateral side. The measurements from the healthy adjacent or similar contralateral skin provides an intraindividual reference measurement that takes into account individual variability of the skin owing to both intrinsic and extrinsic factors. The second EIS measurement is obtained from lesional skin.

## Studies

The EIS diagnostic algorithm was developed based on the EIS measurement results acquired on 751 lesions from 681 patients. All lesions were subsequently excised and the diagnosis histopathologically verified. In this initial trial 2 different algorithms were created and tested.[2] For the first algorithm, data from 40% of the lesions were used for training and 60% for testing. The sensitivity for melanoma was calculated to be 98.1%, for nonmelanoma skin cancer it was 100%, and for dysplastic nevi with severe atypia it was 86.2%. The overall calculated specificity for this first algorithm was 23.6%.

For the second classification algorithm, approximately 55% of the data was used for training and 45% for testing. The observed sensitivity for melanoma was 99.4%, for nonmelanoma skin cancer 98.0%, and dysplastic nevi with severe atypia was 93.8%. The overall observed specificity was 24.5%.[2] The observed sensitivity of the local pathologist (as compared with the dermatopathology panel as gold standard) for melanoma was 86.1%, nonmelanoma skin

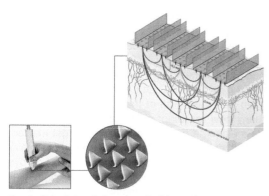

**Fig. 3.** Principle of the electrical impedance spectroscopy measurements at different depths. (*Courtesy of* SciBase, Stockholm, Sweden; with permission.)

cancer 96.9%, and the observed specificity was 92.6%. The sensitivity of the dermatologists pathologist (as compared with the dermatopathology panel as gold standard) was 100% with a specificity of 8.4%.

For the correct interpretation of these results, it is important keep in mind that the lesions included in the study were preselected by the clinician as being suspicious for melanoma, that is, per trial design a clinical sensitivity of

100% and specificity of 0%. A second study confirmed the usefulness of EIS as adjunct diagnostic tool to help clinicians to differentiate between benign and malignant melanocytic skin lesions.

More recently, the results of an international, multicenter, prospective, blinded clinical trial on efficacy and safety of EIS have been published.[1] This trial was conducted in 5 US and 17 European sites that evaluated 2416 lesions in 1951 patients. Of the lesions 2416 evaluated, 1943 were eligible and evaluable and included 112 in situ melanomas, 153 invasive melanomas with a median Breslow thickness of 0.57 mm, 48 basal cell carcinomas, and 7 squamous cell carcinomas.

Similar to the first trial, the lesions included in this study were preselected by the dermatologist as being suspicious for melanoma and were scheduled for excision. To ensure that a broad spectrum of excised lesions will be included in the study, dermatologists were encouraged to enroll a mix of lesions with an even distribution of low, medium, and high pretest probabilities of being melanoma. The exclusion criteria were age younger than 18, melanoma metastasis or recurrent disease, lesions smaller than 2 mm and larger than 20 mm, lesions on acral sites, lesions on hair-bearing areas,

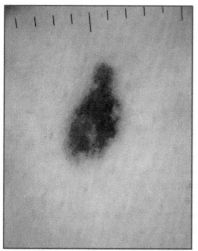

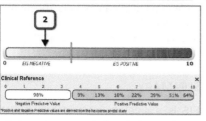

Lesion Description
- Size: 4x6 mm
- Location: Upper back
- Flat lesion
- No evolution

Patient Information
- Female, Age: 36
- No history of MM

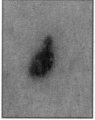

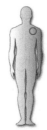

Dermoscopy malignancy grading (0–10): 8

Nevisense EIS score: 2

Histopathology: Benign

**Fig. 4.** Clinical, dermoscopy, and electrical impedance spectroscopy (EIS) score of a benign nevus. MM, malignant melanoma. (*Courtesy of* SciBase, Stockholm, Sweden; with permission.)

lesions on mucosal surfaces, and lesions on areas with other skin disease, such as eczema.[1,2]

For all lesions, EIS measurements and histopathology were performed. Histology was performed by the local dermatopathologist and, in addition, the histopathology slides were also reviewed by a panel of 3 experienced histopathologists who evaluated each lesion independently without knowledge of the histopathology diagnosis rendered by the other pathologists. In the cases of agreement in diagnosis among the experts, that diagnosis was considered as the study's histopathologic gold standard. If there was disagreement among the pathology reviewers on whether the lesion represented a malignancy, the respective slides were submitted to 2 additional experts whose diagnosis was then chosen as the histopathologic gold standard if they reached agreement. In cases of disagreement by the 2 additional reviewers, the corresponding lesion was excluded from the efficacy analysis.

The EIS device calculated a score (range, 0–10) and a dichotomous output (EIS negative or positive) at a fixed cutoff. The fixed threshold was set at 4, that is, scores of less than 4 are EIS negative for malignancy and scores of 4 or greater are EIS positive for malignancy. The dichotomous output was used in this study to calculate the sensitivity and specificity end points with histopathology consensus serving as the gold standard as outlined.

Of the 1943 eligible and evaluable lesions, 265 (13.2%) were melanoma and 55 (2.8%) were nonmelanoma skin cancer. The EIS algorithm correctly identified 256 melanomas and all 55 nonmelanoma skin cancers, yielding an observed sensitivity of 96.6% and 100%, respectively. A total of 157 nevi with severe dysplasia were included, of which the EIS algorithm gave a positive reading for malignancy in 132 cases.

The positive predictive value of the EIS algorithm was 21.1% and the negative predictive value was 98.2%. The EIS algorithm score correlated well with the lesion's degree of histopathology severity. In this study, the observed sensitivity and specificity for melanoma of the local histopathologists was 84.9% and 98.1%, respectively (consensus expert pathologist panel serving as the gold standard). The observed sensitivity for melanoma in situ was 73.2% and this increased to 100% for melanomas with a thickness between T1b-T4 and T2b-T4.

## DISCUSSION

Differentiating melanoma from atypical nevi can be challenging, especially in patients with many atypical nevi. The clinical decision making process is complex and takes into account patient's history, risk factors, analytical analysis of the lesion (ie, ABCDE criteria), differential recognition (ie, outlier lesions), comparative recognition (ie, change over time), and gut feeling.[3] However, even after taking all of these items into account, many nevi are biopsied because of the concern for melanoma and some melanomas get missed. To further assist in differentiating nevi from melanoma requires leveraging technology to improve sensitivity and specificity. These technologies include dermoscopy, reflectance confocal microscopy, and EIS, just to mention a few.

EIS is intended to be used on lesions that are deemed to be suspicious for melanoma based on clinical and dermoscopic examination. In this group of lesions, EIS was able to achieve a high sensitivity (96.6%) for melanoma detection in a cohort of lesions consisting of in situ and early invasive melanoma and dysplastic nevi. The specificity was superior to the clinician's naked eye.[1] The observed sensitivity of the device increased as the thickness of melanoma increased. It is noteworthy that none of the invasive melanomas were missed by the device.

The overall observed specificity for atypical nevi was 34.4%. In other words, approximately one-third of the equivocal lesions submitted for biopsy in the study were accurately identified as benign or negative by EIS and theoretically a biopsy could have been avoided in these lesions. In addition, the high observed negative predictive value of 98 2%, which was equal to the negative predictive value of histology in the study, ensures that few melanomas were inaccurately left unbiopsied.

Although further work is required to determine the ability of EIS to correctly classify other lesions such as lentigines and seborrheic keratosis as benign, in the present study the seborrheic keratoses were classified inaccurately as being malignant by EIS. This observation underscores the importance that EIS should be performed by clinicians trained to correctly recognize seborrheic keratosis, thus preventing them from be evaluated via EIS.

Although the sensitivity for the diagnosis of nonmelanoma skin cancer was 100%, more research is required to determine the efficacy of EIS in diagnosing different subtypes and stages of nonmelanoma skin cancers.

## SUMMARY

EIS is a safe device that has a high sensitivity for detecting skin cancer. The scores provided by EIS may be used in conjunction with the clinical assessment to assist in management decisions.

## REFERENCES

1. Malvehy J, Hauschild A, Curiel-Lewandrowski C, et al. Clinical performance of the Nevisense system in cutaneous melanoma detection: an international, multicentre, prospective and blinded clinical trial on efficacy and safety. Br J Dermatol 2014;171(5): 1099–107.
2. Mohr P, Birgersson U, Berking C, et al. Electrical impedance spectroscopy as a potential adjunct diagnostic tool for cutaneous melanoma. Skin Res Technol 2013;19(2):75–83.
3. Marghoob AA, Scope A. The complexity of diagnosing melanoma. J Invest Dermatol 2009; 129(1):11–3.

# Using Raman Spectroscopy to Detect and Diagnose Skin Cancer In Vivo

Jianhua Zhao, PhD[a,b], Haishan Zeng, PhD[a,b],
Sunil Kalia, MD, MHSc[a,b], Harvey Lui, MD[a,b],*

## KEYWORDS

- Skin cancer • Raman spectroscopy • In vivo • Spectrum
- Imaging-guided confocal Raman spectroscopy

## KEY POINTS

- Raman spectroscopy is a noninvasive optical technique that measures the chemical vibrational modes of molecules within tissue.
- Raman tissue signals are extremely weak and require specialized spectrometers and optical probes to be detected.
- Raman spectroscopy for in vivo clinical applications has been developed as a diagnostic aid for skin cancer.
- Recent clinical studies suggest that Raman spectroscopy may potentially be at least comparable or superior to other diagnostic techniques.

## INTRODUCTION

Skin cancers, including basal cell carcinoma (BCC), squamous cell carcinoma (SCC), and melanoma, are the most common human malignancies. The clinical diagnosis of skin cancers is customarily based on visual inspection followed by invasive biopsy of suspicious lesions. The overall level of accuracy relies heavily on the experience and training of the health care professional.

To aid skin cancer diagnosis, several optical techniques have been proposed, including Raman spectroscopy,[1–4] spectral imaging,[5] optical coherence tomography,[6] and dermoscopy.[7] Raman spectroscopy has now been implemented as a real-time, in vivo tool for use at the bedside, and has been approved in the European Union, Canada, and Australia, but not yet by the US Food and Drug Administration.

Disclosures: The authors and the BC Cancer Agency hold patents for Raman spectroscopy that are licensed to Verisante Technology Inc. This project is financially supported by grants from the Canadian Cancer Society (CCS, grant 015053), the Canadian Institutes of Health Research (CIHR, grant PP2-111527 and MOP130548), the Canadian Dermatology Foundation (CDF), the VGH & UBC Hospital Foundation In It for Life Fund, and the BC Hydro Employee's Community Services (HYDRECS) Fund.
[a] Photomedicine Institute, Department of Dermatology and Skin Science, Vancouver Coastal Health Research Institute, The University of British Columbia, 835 West 10th Avenue, Vancouver, British Columbia V5Z 4E8, Canada; [b] Imaging Unit, Integrative Oncology Department, The BC Cancer Agency Research Center, 675 West 10th Avenue, Vancouver, British Columbia V5Z 1L3, Canada
* Corresponding author. Department of Dermatology and Skin Science, The University of British Columbia, 835 West 10th Avenue, Vancouver, British Columbia V5Z 4E8, Canada.
E-mail address: Harvey.Lui@ubc.ca

Dermatol Clin 35 (2017) 495–504
http://dx.doi.org/10.1016/j.det.2017.06.010
0733-8635/17/© 2017 Elsevier Inc. All rights reserved.

derm.theclinics.com

# WHAT DOES RAMAN SPECTROSCOPY MEASURE?

## What Is the Raman Effect and What Influences It?

The Raman scattering effect was first discovered experimentally by the Indian physicist, C.V. Raman in 1928, and is related to the chemical vibrational modes of molecules. As shown in **Fig. 1**A, almost all of the incoming light photons that reach any molecule are either absorbed or scattered. If a photon is absorbed, its energy is transferred to the molecule, whereas if a photon's path is scattered by the molecule, its energy is conserved, and this scattering event is thus said to be "*elastic*." A very tiny proportion of scattered photons ($\sim 10^{-10}$; ie, 1 of every 10 billion photons) is scattered "*inelastically*," meaning that the energy of the incident photon changes slightly as its path is scattered by the molecule. This minor energy difference between the incident and inelastically scattered photon is known as the Raman effect (or shift) and this energy corresponds to the unique molecular vibrational levels of the scattering molecule. Because photon energy is inversely related to wavelength, the Raman shift also will manifest as a slight color shift for the scattered photon; this color shift requires a highly sensitive spectrometer to detect.

In physics, Raman scattering is governed by several selection rules that are related to molecular vibrations, including symmetric stretching, asymmetric stretching, bending, rocking,

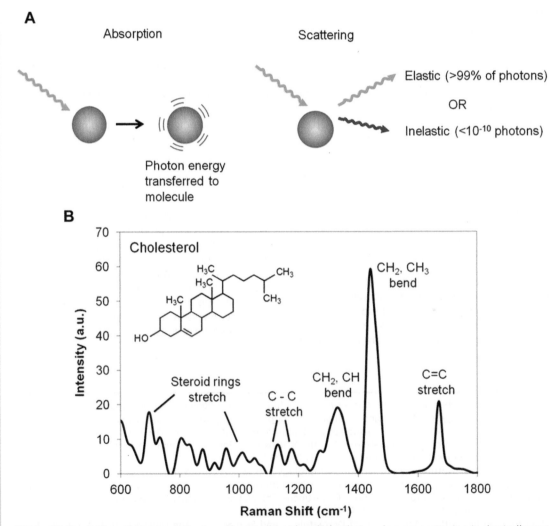

**Fig. 1.** (*A*) Illustration of Raman scattering. Almost all incident light that undergoes scattering is elastically scattered with photon energy being conserved. A very tiny proportion (ie, $10^{-10}$) of scattering occurs inelastically with a small shift in energy known as the Raman effect. (*B*) Raman spectrum for cholesterol showing multiple signal peaks, each corresponding to different molecular bond vibrations.

wagging, and scissoring. These modes involve energy levels corresponding to that of infrared (IR) radiation, and the Raman shift for a molecule is thus related, but not identical to its IR absorption spectrum. Raman spectroscopy and IR absorption spectroscopy are complementary, but for in vivo tissue measurements, Raman spectroscopy is superior to IR absorption spectroscopy. The preferred measurement geometry for IR absorption spectroscopy is a transmission configuration, which is inconvenient or impossible to implement for in vivo applications. In contrast, Raman spectroscopy facilitates a back-scattering/reflection measurement geometry that is ideally suited for in vivo applications. Another practical issue is that the high water content of in vivo tissue exhibits strong IR absorption that overwhelms the IR absorption spectral features of other tissue molecules. Raman spectroscopy shifts the spectral measurements to the visible or near IR wavelength range, which is minimally affected by the presence of water.

As shown in **Fig.** 1B, a Raman spectrum is commonly expressed in intensity as a function of Raman shift, given by $v = 1/\lambda_0 - 1/\lambda$, where $\lambda$ and $\lambda_0$ are the wavelengths of the Raman signal and the excitation light respectively; $v$ is the Raman shift in wavenumbers ($cm^{-1}$), which usually ranges up to 4000 wavenumbers (ie, $cm^{-1}$). The range below 2000 $cm^{-1}$ is often called the fingerprint region, where the Raman signal is abundant and unique for most biological molecules. The region above 2000 $cm^{-1}$ is often called the high-frequency region, consisting of Raman peaks mainly from lipids, proteins, and water. The Raman shift in wavenumbers is an absolute energy difference between the Raman signal and the incident light. To the extent that diseased tissue exhibits differences in molecular composition as compared with normal tissue, Raman spectra will vary between pathologic and healthy states.

Although the existence of the Raman effect has been known since the early twentieth century, the ability to detect these extremely weak, but highly informative optical signals from tissue has only recently been technically feasible.

### What Information Does Raman Provide?

Raman signals are highly dependent on the structure and conformation of biochemical constituents at the molecular level, and therefore are regarded as molecular fingerprints. The Raman shift of a peak indicates a specific vibrational mode within a specific molecule. The Raman intensities of various peaks correspond to the quantity of the molecules within the sample. Therefore, one can quantify and characterize molecules by measuring their Raman intensities and shifts from the recorded spectra.

### HOW DOES RAMAN SCATTERING DIFFER FROM OTHER OPTICAL METHODS FOR DIAGNOSIS; THAT IS, REFLECTANCE, FLUORESCENCE, OPTICAL COHERENCE GATING, AND CONFOCAL TECHNIQUES?

There are 3 basic light-tissue interactions, including absorption, scattering (elastic and inelastic), and fluorescence. All optical methods involving spectroscopy and/or imaging are based on 1 or more of these interactions. Raman is based on the inelastic scattering effect, which is more specific at the molecular level than other techniques. Absorbers (ie, chromophores), scatterers, and fluorophores within skin tissue include the following:

- Skin chromophores include structural proteins and nucleic acids in the UV range; melanin, hemoglobin, and bilirubin in the visible range; and water and fat in the infrared range.
- Elastic optical scattering is mainly caused by refractive index fluctuations. The main elastic scatters in skin include interfaces of cell membranes, nuclei, and collagen fibers.
- Most skin molecules cause inelastic (Raman) optical scattering, such as all types of amino acids, proteins, lipids, and nucleic acids.
- Skin (endogenous) fluorophores include tryptophan, porphyrins, collagen fibers, elastic fibers, keratin fibers, flavins, and nicotinamide adenine dinucleotide.

The most commonly used spectroscopic techniques involve reflectance, fluorescence, or Raman scattering, and are based on recording these optical effects as a function of wavelength. Clinical spectroscopic devices typically assess specific points within tissue, and spectroscopic approaches are usually faster than their imaging counterparts.

Optical imaging techniques can also use reflectance, fluorescence, or Raman scattering to quantify the spatial distribution of these interactions at a specified wavelength or waveband region. For example, standard digital photography records the spatial distribution of elastic scattering and/or absorption by the skin within the visible wavelength range. Dermoscopy is essentially magnified digital imaging with higher resolution than regular digital imaging.

When combined with other techniques, these spectroscopic or imaging techniques can be further refined into different modalities, such as reflectance confocal microscopy, which combines confocal detection with ballistic reflection (ie, single elastic scattering events); optical coherence tomography, which combines coherent gating detection with ballistic reflection; and spectral imaging, which incorporates integrated spectral and spatial information. A brief comparison of these techniques is summarized in **Table 1**.

## RAMAN SPECTROSCOPY OF THE SKIN

A set of typical Raman spectra of human skin cancers and benign skin lesions is shown in **Fig. 2**. The spectra are mathematically normalized to simplify visual comparisons. In general, benign and malignant skin lesions appear to share similar Raman peaks and bands. The prominent Raman bands in the fingerprint region are centered around 855, 936, 1002, 1075, 1271, 1302, 1445, 1655, and 1745 $cm^{-1}$. The spectral resolution of most Raman systems is within

**Table 1**
**Comparative features of major spectroscopic and imaging techniques**

| Techniques | Advantages | Disadvantages |
|---|---|---|
| Dermoscopy | • Based on elastic scattering and absorption<br>• Provides morphologic information of surface<br>• Large field of view<br>• Relatively low cost of system | • Lower resolution<br>• No depth information |
| Raman spectroscopy | • Signatures of biomolecules<br>• Sensitive to biochemical and morphologic changes<br>• No sample preparation<br>• In vivo applications | • Extremely weak signal<br>• System is more expensive than other spectroscopy<br>• Slow in imaging mode |
| Reflectance spectroscopy | • Very strong signal<br>• Fast acquisition<br>• Low cost of system<br>• In vivo applications<br>• Fast in imaging mode | • Depends on scatters and absorbers<br>• Less biochemical information |
| Fluorescence spectroscopy | • Relatively strong signal<br>• Relatively fast acquisition<br>• Relatively low cost of system<br>• *In vivo* applications<br>• Can be used in imaging mode<br>• Contains structural and biochemical information | • Spectra of different fluorophores are broad and often overlapped<br>• Quantitative analysis is difficult |
| Reflectance confocal microscopy | • Based on ballistic reflectance<br>• Out of focus signal is rejected<br>• High horizontal and axial resolution<br>• Horizontal imaging | • Limited field of view<br>• Limited imaging depth<br>• No functional imaging |
| Optical coherence tomography | • Based on ballistic reflectance<br>• Vertical imaging mode<br>• Higher penetration depth than confocal imaging<br>• In vivo applications | • Low horizontal resolution<br>• Lower resolution than confocal imaging<br>• No functional imaging |
| Spectral imaging | • Spectral and spatial information<br>• In vivo applications<br>• Reflectance or fluorescence mode | • System is more expensive<br>• Slower acquisition |
| Raman imaging | • Functional imaging<br>• Provides spatial information of biochemical signatures | • Imaging speed is slow<br>• Ideal for ex vivo applications<br>• System requires more expensive instrumentation to acquire coherent anti-Stokes Raman signals for imaging |

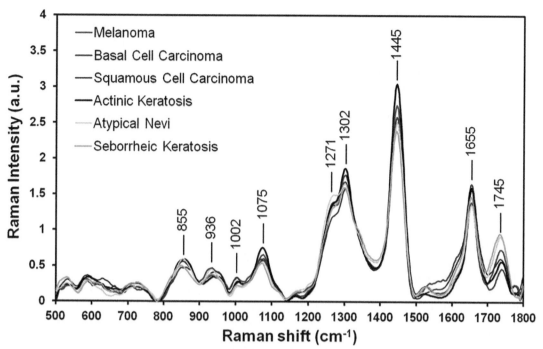

Fig. 2. Typical Raman spectra of skin cancers and benign skin lesions. All the spectra are normalized to their respective areas under the curve in the range 500 to 1800 cm$^{-1}$ to facilitate visual comparison. (*From* Lui H, Zhao J, McLean D, et al. Real-time Raman spectroscopy for in vivo skin cancer diagnosis. Cancer Res 2012;72:2495; with permission.)

4 to 8 cm$^{-1}$. In most situations, the strongest Raman peak in the fingerprint region is located around 1445 cm$^{-1}$, which is assigned to $CH_2$ and $CH_3$ bonds of lipids and proteins in the bending vibrational mode. Another prominent Raman band is around 1655 cm$^{-1}$, which is attributed to keratin protein vibrational modes involving amide I bonds. The 2 overlapping bands around 1271 and 1302 cm$^{-1}$, which are assigned to amide III and a twisting deformation of the $CH_2$ methylene groups of intracellular lipid acyls, respectively, are also typical Raman features of normal skin and skin pathologies. The 2 peaks at 855 cm$^{-1}$ and 936 cm$^{-1}$, assigned to C-C stretching mode, like 2 humps of a camel, are the signatures of collagen type I. The phenylalanine peak around 1002 cm$^{-1}$ is observed in all the pathologies. The region from 1000 to 1150 cm$^{-1}$ contains information about aliphatic hydrocarbon chains. The band around 1745 cm$^{-1}$ is assigned to the C=O stretching mode of the lipid ester, but may have traces of contribution of melanin in vivo.[8] **Fig. 2** also demonstrates that pigmented lesions (melanoma, atypical nevus, and seborrheic keratosis) have higher Raman signals than nonpigmented skin cancers (BCC and SCC, and actinic keratosis) at 1745 cm$^{-1}$.

## HOW TO ASSESS RAMAN SPECTRA

The quality of Raman spectrum can be assessed simply by visual inspection of the typical Raman bands; however, there are no distinctive Raman peaks or bands that can be uniquely assigned to a specific skin pathology by simply visual inspection alone. Therefore, we must rely on more sophisticated statistical methods to extract the diagnostic information, such as partial least squares, principal component general discriminate analysis, neural networks, or support vector machines.[2]

## CLINICAL STUDIES OF RAMAN SPECTROSCOPY

Raman spectroscopy has been used to study dysplasia and cancer in a variety of tissue types besides skin, including lung,[9–12] breast,[13–19] stomach,[20–24] colon,[25–29] cervix,[30–34] oral mucosa,[35] and bladder.[36] All achieved reasonably high sensitivities and specificities.

## RAMAN SPECTROSCOPY IN DERMATOLOGY

Raman spectroscopy was first reported for skin investigation by Edwards and his colleagues in 1992.[37,38] They measured a number of ex vivo skin samples using a Fourier transform Raman (FT-Raman) system and characterized the major Raman peaks for skin samples. It took approximately 30 minutes to acquire a single Raman spectrum using the FT-Raman system at that time.[39] Since then, it has been used for assessment of cosmetic products, monitoring cutaneous drug delivery, and evaluation of skin aging and photoaging.

## Skin Cancer Diagnosis by Ex Vivo Raman Spectroscopy

Earlier studies were focused on ex vivo skin cancer diagnosis using FT-Raman spectroscopy. For example, Gniadecka and colleagues[40] reported the feasibility of FT-Raman spectroscopy for diagnosis of BCC. In this study, they measured 16 BCC and 16 normal skin biopsies by FT-Raman spectrometer excited at 1064 nm, and quantified the difference between BCC and normal skin. In a separate article,[41] the Raman properties of benign and malignant skin biopsies were quantified using an FT-Raman spectrometer. The sample size of this study was small (n = 38), but differences between pathologies were demonstrated among several Raman bands. Several subsequent studies evaluated the diagnosis of melanoma and nonmelanoma skin cancer ex vivo using FT-Raman spectroscopy.[42–44] The largest skin cancer study using FT-Raman to measure ex vivo skin samples (n = 223) included 22 melanomas, 41 pigmented nevi, 48 BCCs, 23 seborrheic keratoses, and 89 normal skin sites. Measurements had an integration time of approximately 7 minutes for each spectrum at 1064-nm excitation, and achieved a sensitivity of 85% and specificity of 99% using a neural network classification model.[42] Recently, Philipsen and colleagues[45] reported that melanoma and BCC diagnosis was independent of skin pigmentation using FT-Raman.

Puppels and colleagues[46–49] developed a confocal microscopic Raman system and measured the Raman properties of different skin layers ex vivo and in vivo. In a confocal configuration, it took approximately 10 seconds to 8 minutes to acquire a single Raman spectrum, which limited its practicality for large-scale studies. Normal skin and BCC skin biopsies were measured ex vivo with an 850-nm laser (12 nodular BCCs and 3 superficial BCCs) and achieved a sensitivity of 100% and specificity of 93%.[50] Another study[51] investigated measured normal and BCC skin samples ex vivo in the high-frequency region with a 720-nm laser (19 BCCs and 9 normal), and demonstrated that Raman spectroscopy in the high-frequency region could also differentiate BCC

from normal tissue with high accuracy. Diagnosis of melanoma ex vivo from melanocytic lesions by FT-Raman spectroscopy in the high-frequency region alone (at 976-nm excitation) has achieved an area under the receiver operator characteristic curve of 0.77.[52] Barriers to the uptake of *ex vivo* Raman measurements in the clinical setting include that the procedure is invasive, the properties of the samples may change after biopsy, and that FT-Raman measurements are time-consuming. Therefore, studies using in vivo Raman measurements with a faster acquisition time are important steps for uptake of this technology at the bedside.

## Skin Cancer Diagnosis In Vivo by Raman Spectroscopy

Technical advances in Raman systems with reduced acquisition times have allowed for in vivo measurements to be collected. Mahadevan-Jansen and her colleagues[53,54] developed a fiber-based confocal Raman system for ex vivo and in vivo skin cancer diagnosis. The integration time of such kind of system is still fairly long (approximately 30 seconds for a single Raman spectrum). They demonstrated that confocal microscopic Raman spectroscopy could be used for skin cancer diagnosis with high diagnostic performance. However, their in vivo study was limited to a small number of cases (9 BCCs, 4 SCCs, 8 inflamed scars, and 21 normal).

We developed a real-time Raman system for skin cancer diagnosis with 785-nm excitation and reduced the spectral acquisition to less than a second.[55,56] A diagram of the system is schematically shown in **Fig. 3**. The hand-held Raman probe is fiber-based so it can access most body sites. During the measurement, the hand-held Raman probe is placed in gentle contact with the skin site without compressing it. This system has been tested for in vivo skin cancer diagnosis.

Recently, we reported the first large-scale clinical study of Raman spectroscopy for in vivo skin cancer diagnosis.[1] It is the first large-scale study to prove that Raman spectroscopy could be a useful clinical tool for in vivo skin cancer diagnosis. In this study, 518 validated lesions were analyzed (including 44 melanoma, 109 BCCs, 47 SCCs, 32 actinic keratosis, 57 atypical nevi, 34 junction nevi, 30 compound nevi, 38 intradermal nevi, 13 blue nevi, and 114 seborrheic keratosis), with each spectrum being measured in less than a second in vivo. The performance of real-time Raman spectroscopy for skin cancer diagnosis is shown in **Fig. 4**. The area under the receiver operating characteristic (ROC) curve is 0.879

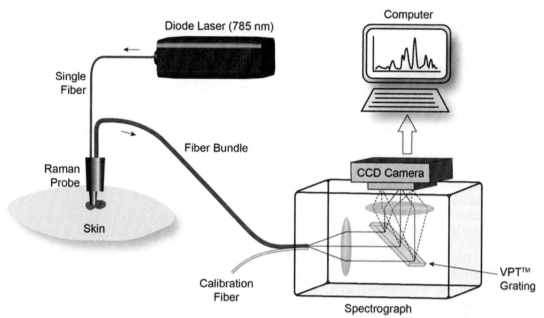

**Fig. 3.** Diagram of real-time in vivo Raman spectrometer system. The hand-held Raman probe is fiber-based so it can access to most of the body sites. The laser is delivered to the probe through a single fiber, and the signal is collected by the probe and delivered to the spectrograph through a fiber bundle. During the measurement, the hand-held Raman probe is placed in gentle contact with the skin site without compressing it. (*From* Lui H, Zhao J, McLean D, et al. Real-time Raman spectroscopy for in vivo skin cancer diagnosis. Cancer Res 2012;72:2493; with permission.)

(95% confidence interval [CI] 0.829–0.929). At a sensitivity level of 0.90, the specificity is as high as 0.64, superior to clinicians and other diagnostic aids.[1] We further validated these findings in a

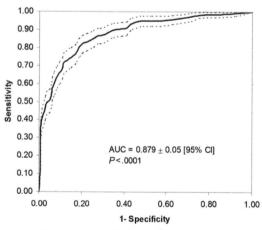

**Fig. 4.** ROC curve of discriminating skin cancers and precancers from benign skin diseases by real-time in vivo Raman spectroscopy. Dashed lines: 95% confidence intervals CIs. The area under the ROC curve (AUC) is 0.879 (95% CI 0.829–0.929). (*From* Lui H, Zhao J, McLean D, et al. Real-time Raman spectroscopy for in vivo skin cancer diagnosis. Cancer Res 2012;72:2496; with permission.)

completely independent study,[57] in which we measured 127 new cases, including 77 cancerous lesions and 50 benign lesions. The diagnostic algorithm generated from the previous study[1] is applied directly to the new cases, and similar diagnostic performance of the new cases is obtained. Recently, we proposed a new wavenumber-selection–based algorithm, thereby focusing on the most discriminative wavebands for diagnosis. The new algorithm improves the diagnostic specificity with high sensitivity levels. For example, the specificity could be improved from 0.64 to 0.75 at a sensitivity level of 0.90.[58]

## How Raman Spectroscopy Is Used in Clinics

In the clinical setting, real-time Raman spectroscopy is meant to be used as an adjunct to conventional diagnostic approaches for lesions suspected of being skin cancer. The clinician holds a Raman probe over the skin lesion and records a spectral measurement with a finger-activated switch. A Raman spectrum is measured within a second. The system does not require the clinician to visually analyze the Raman spectrum itself, but rather the device displays the percentage predicted probability for malignancy for that lesion via an automated internal algorithm analysis of the spectrum. The clinician then uses this predicted risk in combination with his or her visual assessment and/or other diagnostic aids, such as dermoscopy, to make a final decision regarding biopsy.

## RAMAN COMBINED WITH OTHER DIAGNOSTIC METHODS

### Raman Imaging

Conventional Raman imaging measures the spontaneous Raman emission by point or line scanning, which generates a spectral cube that can map the spatial distribution of different Raman signatures.[59] Because each pixel represents a single Raman spectrum, it is so slow that it is applicable only for ex vivo laboratory applications. Advanced techniques for Raman imaging are based on several Raman enhancement techniques, including coherent anti-Stokes Raman scattering and stimulated Raman scattering imaging.[60–62] Both techniques need to use an ultrafast laser (picosecond or femtosecond laser) for excitation. Such systems are more complicated and expensive, and remain investigational.

### Imaging-Guided Confocal Raman Spectroscopy

Confocal Raman spectroscopy incorporates the advantage of confocal microscopy, in which the signals from out-of-the-target areas are rejected. Such spectral systems have been used for skin evaluation,[49,63–65] monitoring cutaneous drug delivery[66] and skin cancer diagnosis.[53,54] In general, 2 separate light sources are used in confocal Raman spectroscopy, with one for confocal imaging and the other for Raman measurement. The targeted area is first located under confocal microscopy and then the imaging mode is turned off to allow for confocal Raman measurement. Such a system is problematic for *in vivo* clinical applications because the measured area may be off the targeted area due to movement of the patient. Recently, we developed an in vivo confocal Raman spectroscopy system under the guidance of reflectance confocal microscopy using a single laser source.[67] The region of interest can be varied from $10 \times 10$ µm to $300 \times 300$ µm. Raman spectra of different skin layers or microstructures can be measured under in vivo confocal microscopy. Such a system could be used to image blood vessels and monitor blood glucose levels. These systems are also investigational.

## SUMMARY

In summary, Raman spectroscopy provides a unique noninvasive bedside tool that captures unique optical signals via molecular vibrations in tissue samples. Raman theory was discovered at the beginning of the twentieth century, but it was not until the past few decades that it has been used to differentiate skin neoplasms. We have provided a brief description of Raman spectroscopy for in vivo skin cancer diagnosis, including the physical principles underlying Raman spectroscopy, its advantages, typical spectra of skin pathologies, and the assessment method for skin cancer diagnosis.

## REFERENCES

1. Lui H, Zhao J, McLean D, et al. Real-time Raman spectroscopy for in vivo skin cancer diagnosis. Cancer Res 2012;72:2491–500.
2. Wang W, Zhao J, Short M, et al. Real-time in vivo cancer diagnosis using Raman spectroscopy. J Biophotonics 2015;8:527–45.
3. Austin LA, Osseiran S, Evans CL. Raman technologies in cancer diagnostics. Analyst 2016;141:476–503.
4. Pence I, Mahadevan-Jansen A. Clinical instrumentation and applications of Raman spectroscopy. Chem Soc Rev 2016;45:1958–79.
5. Tomatis S, Carrara M, Bono A, et al. Automated melanoma detection with a novel multispectral imaging system: results of a prospective study. Phys Med Biol 2005;50:1675.
6. Sattler E, Kästle R, Welzel J. Optical coherence tomography in dermatology. J Biomed Opt 2013; 18:061224.
7. Menzies SW, Bischof L, Talbot H, et al. The performance of solarscan: an automated dermoscopy image analysis instrument for the diagnosis of primary melanoma. Arch Dermatol 2005;141:1388–96.
8. Huang Z, Lui H, Chen XK, et al. Raman spectroscopy of in vivo cutaneous melanin. J Biomed Opt 2004;9:1198–205.
9. Short M, Lam S, McWilliams A, et al. Development and preliminary results of an endoscopic Raman probe for potential in-vivo diagnosis of lung cancers. Opt Lett 2008;33:711–3.
10. Short MA, Lam S, McWilliams AM, et al. Using laser Raman spectroscopy to reduce false positives of autofluorescence bronchoscopies: a pilot study. J Thorac Oncol 2011;6:1206–14.
11. Huang Z, McWilliams A, Lui H, et al. Near-infrared Raman spectroscopy for optical diagnosis of lung cancer. Int J Cancer 2003;107:1047–52.
12. McGregor HC, Short MA, McWilliams A, et al. Real-time endoscopic Raman spectroscopy for in vivo early lung cancer detection. J Biophotonics 2017; 10:98–110.
13. Frank CJ, Mccreery RL, Redd DCB. Raman-spectroscopy of normal and diseased human breast tissues. Anal Chem 1995;67:777–83.

14. Keller MD, Vargis E, de Matos Granja N, et al. Development of a spatially offset Raman spectroscopy probe for breast tumor surgical margin evaluation. J Biomed Opt 2011;16:077006.

15. Barman I, Dingari NC, Saha A, et al. Application of Raman spectroscopy to identify microcalcifications and underlying breast lesions at stereotactic core needle biopsy. Cancer Res 2013;73:3206–15.

16. Haka AS, Volynskaya Z, Gardecki JA, et al. Diagnosing breast cancer using Raman spectroscopy: prospective analysis. J Biomed Opt 2009;14:054023.

17. Haka AS, Shafer-Peltier KE, Fitzmaurice M, et al. Diagnosing breast cancer by using Raman spectroscopy. Proc Natl Acad Sci U S A 2005;102:12371–6.

18. Haka AS, Volynskaya Z, Gardecki JA, et al. In vivo margin assessment during partial mastectomy breast surgery using Raman spectroscopy. Cancer Res 2006;66:3317–22.

19. Redd DCB, Feng ZC, Yue KT, et al. Raman-spectroscopic characterization of human breast tissues—implications for breast-cancer diagnosis. Appl Spectrosc 1993;47:787–91.

20. Teh SK, Zheng W, Ho KY, et al. Diagnostic potential of near infrared Raman spectroscopy in the stomach: differentiating dysplasia from normal tissue. Br J Cancer 2008;98:457–65.

21. Teh SK, Zheng W, Ho KY, et al. Near-infrared Raman spectroscopy for optical diagnosis in the stomach: identification of Helicobacter-pylori infection and intestinal metaplasia. Int J Cancer 2010;126:1920–7.

22. Teh SK, Zheng W, Ho KY, et al. Near-infrared Raman spectroscopy for early diagnosis and typing of adenocarcinoma in the stomach. Br J Surg 2010;97:550–7.

23. Teh SK, Zheng W, Ho KY, et al. Diagnosis of gastric cancer using near-infrared Raman spectroscopy and classification and regression tree techniques. J Biomed Opt 2008;13:034013.

24. Huang Z, Bergholt MS, Zheng W, et al. In vivo early diagnosis of gastric dysplasia using narrow-band image-guided Raman endoscopy. J Biomed Opt 2010;15:037017.

25. Chowdary MVP, Kumar KK, Thakur K, et al. Discrimination of normal and malignant mucosal tissues of the colon by Raman spectroscopy. Photomed Laser Surg 2007;25:269–74.

26. Andrade PO, Bitar RA, Yassoyama K, et al. Study of normal colorectal tissue by FT-Raman spectroscopy. Anal Bioanal Chem 2007;387:1643–8.

27. Widjaja E, Zheng W, Huang Z. Classification of colonic tissue using near-infrared Raman spectroscopy and support vector machines. Int J Oncol 2008;32:653–62.

28. Short MA, Tai IT, Owen D, et al. Using high frequency Raman spectra for colonic neoplasia detection. Opt Express 2013;21:5025–34.

29. Bergholt MS, Lin K, Wang J, et al. Simultaneous fingerprint and high-wavenumber fiber-optic Raman spectroscopy enhances real-time in vivo diagnosis of adenomatous polyps during colonoscopy. J Biophotonics 2015;9:333–42.

30. Mahadevan-Jansen A, Mitchell MF, Ramanujam N, et al. Near-infrared Raman spectroscopy for in vitro detection of cervical precancers. Photochem Photobiol 1998;68:123–32.

31. Utzinger U, Heintzelman DL, Mahadevan-Jansen A, et al. Near-infrared Raman spectroscopy for in vivo detection of cervical precancers. Appl Spectrosc 2001;55:955–9.

32. Duraipandian S, Zheng W, Ng J, et al. Near-infrared-excited confocal Raman spectroscopy advances in vivo diagnosis of cervical precancer. J Biomed Opt 2013;18:67007.

33. Robichaux-Viehoever A, Kanter E, Shappell H, et al. Characterization of Raman spectra measured in vivo for the detection of cervical dysplasia. Appl Spectrosc 2007;61:986–93.

34. Mo J, Zheng W, Low JJ, et al. High wavenumber Raman spectroscopy for in vivo detection of cervical dysplasia. Anal Chem 2009;81:8908–15.

35. Guze K, Pawluk HC, Short M, et al. Pilot study: Raman spectroscopy in differentiating premalignant and malignant oral lesions from normal mucosa and benign lesions in humans. Head Neck 2015;37:511–7.

36. Draga ROP, Grimbergen MCM, Vijverberg PLM, et al. In vivo bladder cancer diagnosis by high-volume Raman spectroscopy. Anal Chem 2010;82:5993–9.

37. Barry BW, Edwards HGM, Williams AC. Fourier transform Raman and infrared vibrational study of human skin: assignment of spectral bands. J Raman Spectrosc 1992;23:641–5.

38. Williams AC, Edwards HGM, Barry BW. Fourier transform Raman spectroscopy: a novel application for examining human stratum corneum. Int J Pharm 1992;81:R11–4.

39. Fendel S, Schrader B. Investigation of skin and skin lesions by NIR-FT-Raman spectroscopy. Fresenius J Anal Chem 1998;360:609–13.

40. Gniadecka M, Wulf HC, Mortensen NN, et al. Diagnosis of basal cell carcinoma by Raman spectroscopy. J Raman Spectrosc 1997;28:125–9.

41. Gniadecka M, Wulf HC, Nielsen OF, et al. Distinctive molecular abnormalities in benign and malignant skin lesions: studies by Raman spectroscopy. Photochem Photobiol 1997;66:418–23.

42. Gniadecka M, Philipsen PA, Sigurdsson S, et al. Melanoma diagnosis by Raman spectroscopy and neural networks: structure alterations in proteins and lipids in intact cancer tissue. J Invest Dermatol 2004;122:443–9.

43. Gniadecka M, Nielsen OF, Wulf HC. Water content and structure in malignant and benign skin tumours. Journal of Molecular Structure 2003;661-662:405–10.

44. Sigurdsson S, Philipsen PA, Hansen LK, et al. Detection of skin cancer by classification of Raman spectra. IEEE Trans Biomed Eng 2004;51:1784–93.

45. Philipsen PA, Knudsen L, Gniadecka M, et al. Diagnosis of malignant melanoma and basal cell carcinoma by in vivo NIR-FT Raman spectroscopy is independent of skin pigmentation. Photochem Photobiol Sci 2013;12:770–6.

46. Caspers PJ, Jacobsen ADT, Lucassen GW, et al. Raman microspectroscopy of human skin. In: Carmona P, Navarro R, Hernanz A, editors. Spectroscopy of Biological Molecules: Modern Trends. Netherlands: Springer; 1997. p. 453–4.

47. Caspers PJ, Lucassen GW, Wolthuis R, et al. In vitro and in vivo Raman spectroscopy of human skin. Biospectroscopy 1998;4:S31–9.

48. Bakker Schut TC, Witjes MJ, Sterenborg HJ, et al. In vivo detection of dysplastic tissue by Raman spectroscopy. Anal Chem 2000;72:6010–8.

49. Caspers PJ, Lucassen GW, Carter EA, et al. In vivo confocal Raman microspectroscopy of the skin: noninvasive determination of molecular concentration profiles. J Invest Dermatol 2001;116:434–42.

50. Nijssen A, Schut TCB, Heule F, et al. Discriminating basal cell carcinoma from its surrounding tissue by Raman spectroscopy. J Invest Dermatol 2002;119:64–9.

51. Nijssen A, Maquelin K, Santos LF, et al. Discriminating basal cell carcinoma from perilesional skin using high wave-number Raman spectroscopy. J Biomed Opt 2007;12:034004.

52. Santos GB, Medeiros IS, Fellows CE, et al. Composite depth of cure obtained with QTH and LED units assessed by microhardness and micro-Raman spectroscopy. Oper Dent 2007;32:79–83.

53. Lieber CA, Majumder SK, Ellis DL, et al. In vivo non-melanoma skin cancer diagnosis using Raman microspectroscopy. Lasers Surg Med 2008;40:461–7.

54. Lieber CA, Majumder SK, Billheimer D, et al. Raman microspectroscopy for skin cancer detection in vitro. J Biomed Opt 2008;13:024013.

55. Zhao J, Lui H, McLean DI, et al. Integrated real-time Raman system for clinical in vivo skin analysis. Skin Res Technol 2008;14:484–92.

56. Huang Z, Zeng H, Hamzavi I, et al. Rapid near-infrared Raman spectroscopy system for real-time in vivo skin measurements. Opt Lett 2001;26:1782–4.

57. Zhao J, Lui H, McLean D, et al. Real-time Raman spectroscopy for noninvasive skin cancer detection—preliminary results. 30th Annual International Conference of the IEEE Engineering in Medicine and Biology Society. Vancouver, Canada, August 20-24, 2008. vols. 1–8. p. 3107–9.

58. Zhao J, Zeng H, Kalia S, et al. Wavenumber selection based analysis in Raman spectroscopy improves skin cancer diagnostic specificity. Analyst 2016;141:1034–43.

59. Klein K, Gigler AM, Aschenbrenner T, et al. Label-free live-cell imaging with confocal Raman microscopy. Biophys J 2012;102:360–8.

60. Evans CL, Xie XS. Coherent anti-Stokes Raman scattering microscopy: chemical imaging for biology and medicine. Annu Rev Anal Chem (Palo Alto Calif) 2008;1:883–909.

61. Evans CL, Potma EO, Puoris' haag M, et al. Chemical imaging of tissue in vivo with video-rate coherent anti-Stokes Raman scattering microscopy. Proc Natl Acad Sci U S A 2005;102:16807–12.

62. Saar BG, Freudiger CW, Reichman J, et al. Video-rate molecular imaging in vivo with stimulated Raman scattering. Science 2010;330:1368–70.

63. Caspers PJ, Lucassen GW, Bruining HA, et al. Automated depth-scanning confocal Raman microspectrometer for rapid in vivo determination of water concentration profiles in human skin. J Raman Spectrosc 2000;31:813–8.

64. Caspers PJ, Lucassen GW, Puppels GJ. Combined in vivo confocal Raman spectroscopy and confocal microscopy of human skin. Biophys J 2003;85:572–80.

65. Caspers PJ, Lucassen GW, Wolthuis R, et al. In vivo Raman spectroscopy of human skin: determination of the composition of natural moisturizing factor. Biomedical Applications of Raman Spectroscopy, Proc. SPIE 1999;3608:99–102.

66. Caspers PJ, Williams AC, Carter EA, et al. Monitoring the penetration enhancer dimethyl sulfoxide in human stratum corneum in vivo by confocal Raman spectroscopy. Pharm Res 2002;19:1577–80.

67. Wang H, Lee AMD, Lui H, et al. A method for accurate in vivo micro-Raman spectroscopic measurements under guidance of advanced microscopy imaging. Sci Rep 2013;3:1890.

# High-Frequency Ultrasound Examination in the Diagnosis of Skin Cancer

Robert L. Bard, MD

## KEYWORDS

- Malignant melanoma • Nonmelanoma skin cancer • Ultrasound guidance • 3D Doppler sonography
- Image guided treatment • Sentinel node biopsy

## KEY POINTS

- Sonographic tumor depth evaluation has 99% histopathologic correlation.
- Melanoma metastatic potential is proportional to vessel density of neovascularity as measured by Doppler histogram analysis.
- Intransit and nonpalpable locoregional metastases can be detected with 3-dimensional image reconstruction.
- Three-dimensional mapping of nerves and arteries optimizes preoperative planning.
- Image-guided biopsy and treatments are cost effective and reduce morbidity.

## INTRODUCTION

Today's health conscious society means adults routinely seek reassurance about suspicious skin lesions. Diagnostic ultrasound examinations can accurately and rapidly differentiate between epidermal, subdermal, and subcutaneous tissues in real time. This procedure may help to identify lesions invisible to the spatially restricted human eye. The high resolution and low cost of today's ultrasonographic equipment allow this modality to be used readily in an outpatient office setting.

The accuracy of ultrasonography in the epidermis, dermis, and subcutaneous tissues is both operator and equipment dependent. Standard 2-dimensional linear sonograms at 40 to 100 MHz image the epidermis. Probes using 15-to 22-MHz image the epidermis and dermis, including the adjacent tissues 1 to 2 cm deep to the basal dermal layer. Real time 3-dimensional (3D/4D) probes at 16 to 20 MHz using broadband technologies provide high resolution of these structures to a 4- to 7-cm depth in seconds. Today's high-resolution equipment is widely available as imaging technology.

## EVOLUTION OF DIAGNOSTIC ULTRASOUND IMAGING

Diagnostic ultrasound examination has been used on the skin and subcutaneous tissues for more than 25 years in Europe and Japan. The technology has evolved from its original use in cyst detection with B scans[1] to its present use for cancer detection using 3D imaging to detect in-transit metastases. Additionally, in vivo flow velocity analysis can now be used to detect melanoma vessel density and analyze tumor microvascularity at 10 micron imaging.[2] Experimental photo and laser acoustic technologies are also currently being studied in animal research. This article provides a basic overview of skin imaging applications. A more in-depth review of dermal ultrasonography may be found elsewhere in the literature.[3]

Bard Cancer Center, 121 East 60th Street, New York, NY 10022, USA
*E-mail address:* rbard@cancerscan.com

Dermatol Clin 35 (2017) 505–511
http://dx.doi.org/10.1016/j.det.2017.06.011
0733-8635/17/© 2017 Elsevier Inc. All rights reserved.

## HOW THE EXAMINATION IS PERFORMED

The application of ultrasonography depends on the area examined and equipment needed for specific diagnosis. All probes require gel contact with the skin and scan duration is typically proportional to the type of probe and examiner's experience. Real-time imaging by a trained physician allows simultaneous picture generation and interpretation to occur within minutes. Routine B scan units require operator-dependent probe motion in 2 planes to obtain orthogonal images. The 3D imaging systems are operator independent because the probe is held steady over the area of interest and electronics scan a 4 × 4-cm area in 6 seconds. Patient motion rarely degrades the images owing to the rapid scan rate. Transducer size is matched to scan areas or can be focused to limited facial regions such as the nose. Three-dimensional imaging of ear and nose cartilage is also available with specialized probes. Lesions can be echogenic or hyperechoic (many internal echoes), such as hemorrhagic areas, echo poor or hypoechoic (few internal echoes), and echo free (no internal echoes), which are usually found in fluid, such as cysts.

## ULTRASOUND EVALUATION OF DERMAL LESIONS

The incidence of melanoma and nonmelanoma skin cancer are both increasing. Earlier detection discovers smaller lesions where focal nonsurgical treatment may be preferred to standard operative techniques, which may limit potential long-term and postoperative side effects. Ultrasound examination permits rapid measurement of skin thickness, fat tissue depth, and fascial integrity. Medical imaging maps arteries, veins, and nerves, which provides preoperative landmarks that can reduce the risk of postoperative bleeding and nerve damage (**Fig. 1**). Image-guided treatment may also decrease the risk of postoperative disfigurement. Interval scans may also be used to track and assess lesions with low aggressive potential.

## DIAGNOSTIC APPLICATIONS FOR NONMELANOMA SKIN CANCER

Clinical diagnosis is the primary modality used to identify nonmelanoma skin cancer; however, visual diagnosis alone cannot determine tumor depth. Imaging allows preoperative mapping of a lesion, which may alert the surgeon to the depth or subclinical extent of a lesion. This information allows surgical planning, which can help to limit the number of stages required and allow for preoperative planning to identify optimal techniques for surgical closure. The presence of coexisting benign disease, such as seborrheic hyperplasia or peritumor inflammatory reaction, may falsely lead to a wider excision or inaccurate biopsy conclusions.

Of basal cell carcinomas, 85% develop in the head and neck, showing a predilection for thin skin, such as the nose, lips, or eyelids. The various shaped probe constructions allow diagnostic evaluation of nearly all locations including external ear compartments (**Fig. 2**). Although most basal cell carcinomas lesions appear as well-defined, oval, echo-poor masses, lesions that may have a higher aggressive potential may also appear as hyperechoic spots.

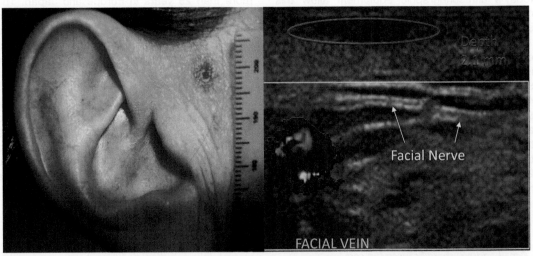

**Fig. 1.** Basal cell carcinoma echo-poor lesion (*circle*) 2.1 mm deep located 5 mm from the facial nerve (*arrows*) and 7 mm from temporal vein (*blue*).

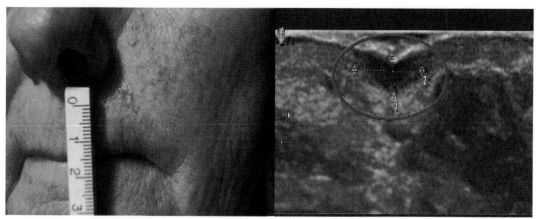

**Fig. 2.** Basal cell carcinoma (*red circle*) echo-poor mass in nasolabial groove imaged with small transducer to improve contact depth measurement of 1.5 mm.

Identification of these foci is useful because neovascularity is less than that in other cancers.[4] Indeed, the appearance of tortuous vessels suggests squamous cell carcinoma, Merkel cell carcinoma, or metastatic tumor. The depth correlation between ultrasonography and histology is excellent,[5] which allows for better preoperative planning (**Fig. 3**).

Squamous cell carcinoma presents as a hypoechoic lesion with irregular borders. Because the thickness or depth of invasion is an important predictor of metastases, the lesion should be followed along its entire course. Extra care is taken to find locoregional metastases and ultrasound examination of the liver and regional nodes may be performed simultaneously. The vascular pattern is increased diffusely throughout the entire mass as opposed to basal cell carcinomas, where the neovascularity is less prominent and often at the bottom of the lesion. Vascular mapping for major feeders with 3D ultrasonography is useful owing to the possibility of widespread penetration of the lesion (**Fig. 4**).

## UNCOMMON DERMAL MALIGNANCIES

Dermatofibrosarcoma protuberans demonstrates a hypoechoic pattern that propagates horizontally and may project into the fascial or muscular layers. Merkel cell carcinoma presents as an echo-poor, ill-defined area. Lymphoma cell varieties have mixed echo patterns (the echo poorones may be mistaken for fluid collections) and variable vascularity. Increased neovascularity is noted in cases with patients on immunosuppressants. Sarcomas are echo poor, except where

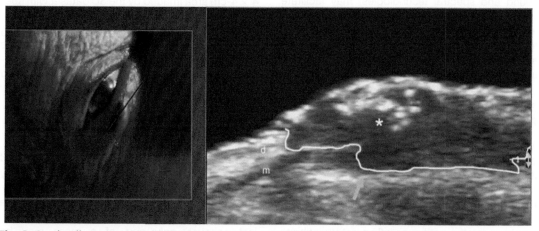

**Fig. 3.** Basal cell carcinoma echo-poor mass with involvement of the orbicularis oculus muscle (m). Tumor (*asterisk*) echogenic foci signifies increased aggression and invades the dermis (d) and muscle layer (m) into the fat (*arrow*).

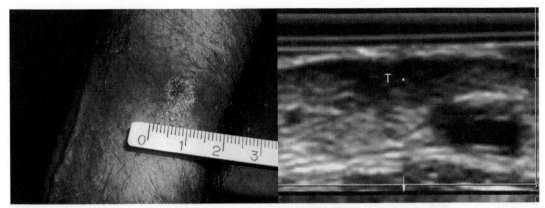

**Fig. 4.** Squamous cell cancer (T) echo-poor mass 2 mm from vein. Note the venous valves as linear white structures (*red arrows*).

internal necrosis and hemorrhage occur. The presence of intact fat–fascial boundaries portends a better prognosis.

## STAGING OF NONMELANOMA SKIN CANCER

Ultrasound imaging accurately measures tumor diameter in all axes, blood flow within and adjacent to the lesion, and the presence of deep layer involvement, including nonpalpable satellites in subcutaneous locations. This staging additionally has the potential to streamline Mohs surgery and provides 1-stage treatment, decreasing the recurrence rate and improving cosmetic outcome.

## MELANOCYTIC LESIONS

Ultrasound screening is well-tolerated and can be highly accurate in the diagnosis of melanocytic skin lesions. The finding of a subclinical metastatic focus near the lesion (provided by newer ultrasound and spectral technologies) may facilitate the physician's decision to pursue further histologic evaluation. Additionally, advanced knowledge of lesion borders, volume, and depth from the skin surfaces could allow for tissue conservation and improved aesthetic outcomes.

## PRIMARY CUTANEOUS MALIGNANT MELANOMA

Melanoma appears as a fusiform, well-defined, echo-poor lesion. At frequencies below 14 MHz, it may appear echo free in a similar fashion to lymphoma owing to the densely packed homogeneous cell architecture (**Fig. 5**). Melanomas less than 0.4 mm often give a false-negative examination because the peritumor inflammatory infiltrate may falsely increase the imaged tumor depth.[6,7] Primary cutaneous melanomas commonly appear

hypervascular.[8–11] Contrast-enhanced ultrasound imaging is the optimal modality to observe arteriovenous shunting and measure Doppler peak systolic and resistance indices. Assessment of angiogenesis also correlates with metastatic potential.[1,12,13] Flow signals can be seen at the tumor base and, less frequently, in the lateral margins. This helps to differentiate melanoma from verruca, where the vascular tree is located centrally and extends to the surface.[14–16] Histogram vessel density analysis has not been reported in the dermal literature, but it is widely used in the evaluation of other malignant tumors.[17–23]

## STAGING OF MALIGNANT MELANOMA

Primary melanoma vascular lesions generally have locoregional vascular metastases, revealing a tissue signature of similar neovascular findings to the original cutaneous disease. Satellite lesions and in-transit metastases are definable within the 4 × 4-cm area imaged by the 3D dataset with specific appearance described as a "tail sign" (**Fig. 6**). Histogram analysis of 99 metastatic foci including 18 melanomas presented at the 2015 Journees Francaises de Radiologie and at the 2016 International Society of Dermatologic Surgery noted vessel density correlated with the Breslow classification.

## IMAGE-GUIDED BIOPSY

New computer programs use nanotechnology and cybernetic modalities for image-guided biopsy and treatment options. Using 3D Doppler ultrasonography, the physician manually targets the area of highest tumor neovascularity. This is critical because only part of a mass may be cancerous and missed on nontargeted punch biopsies. The fusion of MRI with ultrasound imaging

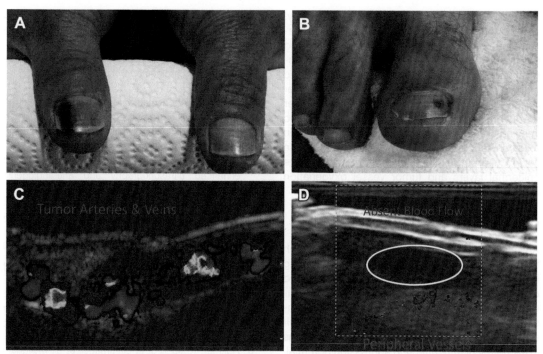

**Fig. 5.** Pigmented lesions. (*A*) Vertical area thumbnail. (*C*) Doppler imaging showing arteriovenous fistulae below nail plate characteristic of melanoma. (*B*) Vertical area toe nail of soccer player. A<B<C (*D*) Doppler imaging showing avascular region consistent with hematoma (*dotted square* indicates field of blood flow imaged).

permits image-guided biopsies sparing adjacent neurovascular bundles, allowing customized ultrasound-guided biopsies to be performed under local anesthesia.

## MELANOMA-RELATED SENTINEL LYMPH NODE BIOPSY

Tumor depth guides appropriate performance of regional nodal lymph node biopsy. Current guidelines suggest that a thickness of greater than 1 mm

reinforces the operative decision for sentinel lymph node biopsy. Ultrasound imaging has the potential to identify sentinel node involvement beyond micrometastases.

## COMPARISON WITH OTHER NONINVASIVE TECHNOLOGIES

In some clinical situations, ultrasound imaging compared favorably with other technologies. Multispectral imaging, optical coherence

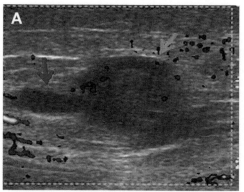
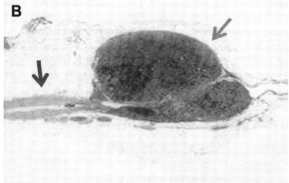

**Fig. 6.** Metastatic melanoma to lymph node. (*A*) Abnormal subcutaneous echo-poor lymph node with echo-poor extension indicated tumor in the lymphatic channel. (*B*) Pathology specimen—lymph duct (*red arrow*) node (*blue arrow*).

tomography, Reflectance Confocal Microscopy, and dermoscopy are limited by depth of penetration, operator experience, availability, and diagnostic specificity.[24] Spectroscopy using electrical impedance, Raman analysis, and proteomic mass are newer procedures currently under investigation (reviewed in this issue). Higher resolution technologies such as photoacoustic imaging and multiphoton analysis used in research laboratories are not clinically available yet, but promise unparalleled imaging of the epidermal layers and tumor vessel oxygenation measurements.

## FUTURE DEVELOPMENTS

Advances in ultrasound imaging include ultrahigh frequency probes from 20 to 100 MHz providing image resolution up to 30 microns and ultrasound contrast agents allowing real-time imaging of tumor neovascularity. Histopathology has demonstrated tumors not only vary markedly over their surface volume in appearance, but have variations in microvasculature affecting aggression potential. Tumor immunohistochemical markers show a strong correlation with tumor neovascularity with subharmonic contrast ultrasound imaging.[25] Three-dimensional ultrasound imaging quantifies vessel density in different quadrants improving targeting. Contrast bubble imaging is not yet approved by the US Food and Drug Administration for the skin, but may add new dimensions in assessment of treatment by monitoring quantitative changes in tumor vessel density.

## SUMMARY

Portable-high resolution ultrasonography now available distinguishes vascular lesions from nonvascular masses. Tumor depth can be measured quickly and locoregional metastases can be accurately observed. Additionally, preoperative imaging may identify cartilage or neural invasion and shorten Mohs surgery and complementary treatments. As ultrasound becomes more mainstream in skin cancer diagnosis and management, a better understanding of the benefits of this technology may occur.

## REFERENCES

1. Lassau N, Spatz A, Avril MF, et al. Value of high frequency US for preoperative assessment of skin tumors. Radiographics 1997;17:1559–65.
2. Errico J, Pierre S, Pezet Y, et al. Ultrafast ultrasound localization microscopy for deep super-resolution vascular imaging. Nature 2015;527:499–502.
3. Wortsman X, Holm EA, Wulf HC, et al. Real time spatial compound imaging of the skin. Skin Res Technol 2004;10:23–31.
4. Wortsman X. Sonography of facial cutaneous basal cell carcinoma. J Ultrasound Med 2013; 32:567–72.
5. Bobadilla F, Wortsman X, Munoz C, et al. Pre-surgical high resolution ultrasound of facial basal cell carcinoma: correlation with histology. Cancer Imaging 2008;8:163–72.
6. Lassau N, Chami L, Chebil M, et al. Dynamic contrast enhanced ultrasonography and anti-angiogenic treatments. Discover Med 2011;11:18–24.
7. Restreppo CS, Ocazionex D. Kaposi's sarcoma: imaging overview. Semin Ultrasound CT MR 2011;32: 456–69.
8. Tacke J, Haagen G, Horstein O, et al. Clinical relevance of sonographically derived tumour thickness in malignant melanoma. Br J Dermatol 1995;132: 209–14.
9. Guitera P, Li PX, Crotty K, et al. Melanoma histological Breslow thickness predicted by 75MHz sonography. Br J Dermatol 2008;159:364–9.
10. Hoffman K, Jung J, el Gammal S, et al. Malignant melanoma in 20 MHz B-scan sonography. Dermatology 1992;185:49–55.
11. Catalano O, Siani A. Cutaneous melanoma: role of ultrasound in the assessment of locoregional spread. Curr Probl Diagn Radiol 2010;39:30–6.
12. Lassau N, Mercier S, Koscielny S, et al. Prognostic value of high frequency sonography and color Doppler for preoperative assessment of melanomas. Am J Roentgenol 1999;172:457–61.
13. Lassau N, Koscielny S, Avril MF, et al. Prognostic value of angiogenesis evaluated by high frequency and Doppler ultrasound for preoperative assessment of melanomas. Am J Roentgenol 2002;178: 1547–51.
14. Nicolaidou E, Mikrova A, Antoniou C, et al. Advances in Merkel cell carcinoma pathogenesis and management. Br J Dermatol 2012;166:16–21.
15. Pileri A Jr, Patrizi A, Agostinelli C, et al. Primary cutaneous lymphomas: a reprisal. Semin Diagn Pathol 2011;28:214–33.
16. Galper SL, Smith BD, Wilson LD. Diagnosis and management of mycosis fungoides. Oncology (Williston Park) 2010;24:491–501.
17. Bard R. Advances in image guided oncologic treatment. J Targ Ther Cancer 2016;1:52–6.
18. Music MM, Hertl K, Kadivec M, et al. Preoperative ultrasound with 15 MHz probe reliably differentiates between melanoma thicker and thinner than 1 mm. J Eur Acad Dermatol Venereol 2010;24: 1105–8.
19. Rossi CR, Mocellin S, Scagnet B, et al. The role of preoperative ultrasound in detecting lymph-node metastases before sentinel node

biopsy in patients with melanoma. J Surg Oncol 2003;83:80–4.

20. Van Rijk MC, Teertstra HJ, Peterse JL, et al. Ultraso-nography and fine needle aspiration cytology in the preoperative evaluation of patients with melanoma eligible for sentinel node biopsy. Ann Surg Oncol 2006;13:1511–6.

21. Ulrich J, van Akooi AC, Eggermont AM, et al. New developments in melanoma: utility of ultrasound im-aging (initial staging). Expert Rev Anticancer Ther 2011;11:1693–701.

22. Voit C, van Akooi AC, Schafer G, et al. Ultrasound morphology criteria predict metastatic disease of the sentinel nodes in patients with melanoma. J Clin Oncol 2010;28:847–52.

23. Catalano O. Critical analysis of the ultrasound criteria for diagnosing lymph node metastases in patients with cutaneous melanoma. J Ultrasound Med 2011;30:547–60.

24. Que SK, Grant-Kels JM, Longo C, et al. Basics of confocal microscopy and the complexity of diag-nosing skin tumors. Dermatol Clin 2016;34:367–75.

25. Gupta A, Forsberg M, Dulin K, et al. Comparing quantitate immunohistochemical markers of angio-genesis to contrast enhanced subharmonic imag-ing. J Ultrasound Med 2016;35:1839–47.

# Proteomic Mass Spectrometry Imaging for Skin Cancer Diagnosis

Rossitza Lazova, MD[a],*, Erin H. Seeley, PhD[b]

## KEYWORDS

- Mass spectrometry • Skin cancer • Melanoma • Atypical melanocytic neoplasm
- Mass spectrometry imaging • Spitzoid melanoma • Atypical Spitzoid neoplasm
- Atypical Spitzoid tumor

## KEY POINTS

- Mass spectrometry imaging studies the proteome and identifies molecular signatures comprising a unique combination of 5 to 20 proteins that enable a specific diagnosis of cancer or disease.
- There are proteomic differences between the melanocytic cells of benign nevi and malignant melanomas, which can be identified by mass spectrometry imaging.
- This technology may assist in the classification of diagnostically challenging melanocytic lesions.
- Mass spectrometry imaging diagnosis of atypical Spitzoid neoplasms seems to predict the clinical outcome better than histopathology and is strongly associated with aggressive clinical behavior.
- Mass spectrometry analysis using a proteomic signature may improve the diagnosis and prediction of outcome/risk stratification for patients with atypical Spitzoid neoplasms and other types of challenging melanocytic lesions.

## INTRODUCTION

Histopathologic examination is currently the gold standard for the diagnosis of melanocytic lesions. However, some problematic cases show overlapping features of both nevi and melanomas. One of the most difficult areas in dermatopathology is distinguishing Spitz nevi from Spitzoid melanomas using current histopathologic criteria.[1–4] Diagnostically challenging cases that show features of both Spitz nevi and Spitzoid melanomas are termed atypical Spitzoid neoplasms. It has been shown in several studies that it can be difficult to predict the clinical behavior of atypical Spitzoid neoplasms from assessment of histopathologic features. The interobserver reproducibility among pathologists for the diagnosis of these tumors is generally poor.[1–5]

Mass spectrometry imaging can be successfully used for skin cancer diagnosis, particularly for the diagnosis of challenging melanocytic lesions. Mass spectrometry imaging analysis is a bioanalytical method for identifying the nature and spatial distribution of biomolecules, including peptides and proteins, DNA segments, lipids, and metabolites, from tissue samples. It has been used to determine the molecular signatures of various types of cancer and other diseases.[6–8] Molecular signatures usually present as a unique combination of 5 to 20 proteins and enable a specific diagnosis.[9] Protein and peptide analysis is superior to gene expression analysis, because it represents the functional state of the disease or tumor rather than the

Disclosures: The authors have nothing to disclose.
[a] California Skin Institute, Department of Pathology, 2420 Samaritan Drive, San Jose, CA 95124, USA; [b] Protea Biosciences, Inc, 1311 Pineview Drive, Suite 501, Morgantown, WV 26505, USA
* Corresponding author.
E-mail address: drlazova@caskin.com

derm.theclinics.com

potential risk of developing it. Furthermore, post-translational modification is thus also considered.

## Methodology

Formalin-fixed, paraffin-embedded 5-μm-thick consecutive tissue sections from each patient are used for mass spectrometry analysis. The first section is placed on a charged slide for mass spectrometry imaging (**Fig. 1**A). The following consecutive section is stained with hematoxylin and eosin (see **Fig. 1**B). A targeted approach is used, in which only discrete areas within a tissue section are analyzed. A dermatopathologist selects and marks these areas, which are 100 μm in diameter (see **Fig. 1**B). On average, 20 different areas containing only melanocytes without admixed dermis or epidermis are marked for each case (see **Fig. 1**B). Many different samples can be analyzed in 1 experiment (see **Fig. 1**C). Images of stained and unstained sections are merged and coordinates of annotations are determined (see **Fig. 1**D). Trypsin and matrix are applied after the

sections are deparaffinized (see **Fig. 1**E) and mass spectra are obtained (see **Fig. 1**F).

The mass spectral profile is acquired for each of the areas of interest (**Fig. 2**). The spectra are then loaded into a software for advanced statistical analysis, visualization, and interpretation of mass spectrometry imaging data. The spectra are baseline corrected, normalized, and peaks are picked and aligned. The samples are sorted into training and validation sets. Hypothesis testing and discriminative m/z (mass to charge ratio) value analysis (receiver operator characteristic curve) are performed on the training set. A linear discriminant analysis classification algorithm is generated and validated on a validation set.

## Application of Mass Spectrometry Imaging in the Diagnosis of Challenging Melanocytic Lesions

### Atypical Spitzoid neoplasms

In a recent mass spectrometry imaging study, we identified differences on the proteomic level

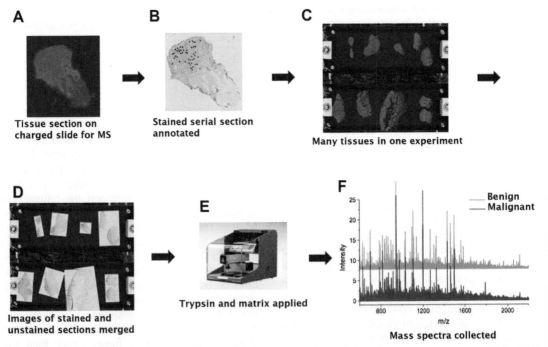

**Fig. 1.** (*A*) An unstained 5 μm-thick tissue section placed on a charged slide for mass spectrometry (MS). (*B*) A consecutive serial section is stained for hematoxylin and eosin. The blue dots in the superficial portion of the lesion represent the areas of pure melanocytic component chosen by the dermatopathologist for mass spectrometric analysis. Additional melanocytic areas colored in red have also been selected to compare differences between the proteomic composition of melanocytes in the superficial and deep portions of the lesion. (*C*) Two adjacent charged slides for mass spectrometry analysis containing 8 separate cases to be analyzed. (*D*) The images of the hematoxylin and eosin–stained sections and unstained sections are merged and this image is used to guide data acquisition for mass spectrometry analysis. (*E*) Trypsin and matrix are applied to the tissue in preparation for mass spectrometry analysis. (*F*) Mass spectra are collected, which show differences in the proteins from the melanocytic components of the benign nevi (*green*) and malignant melanoma (*red*).

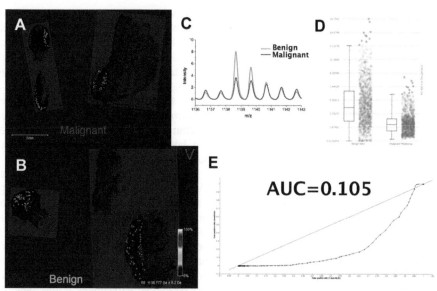

**Fig. 2.** Tryptic peptide at m/z (mass to charge ratio) 1138.8 shows statistically significant differential expression in malignant melanomas and benign nevi. Mass spectrometry images of the peptide showing low intensity in malignant melanomas (*A*) and higher intensity in benign nevi (*B*). (*C*) Average spectra from benign nevi (*green*) and malignant melanomas (*red*). The peptide has 2-fold higher intensity in benign nevi than in malignant melanoma. (*D*) Box and whiskers plot of distributions of the intensity of the peptide at m/z 1138.8 showing complete separation of the boxes (1 standard deviation from the mean). (*E*) Receiver operator characteristic curve for the peptide at m/z 1138.8. The area under the curve (AUC) is 0.105, indicating that this peptide can classify the two groups with 89.5% specificity.

between Spitz nevi and Spitzoid melanomas.[10] Five peptides, comprising a specific proteomic signature, were differentially expressed by the melanocytic component of Spitz nevi and Spitzoid melanomas in formalin-fixed, paraffin-embedded tissue samples. In a subsequent study, we sought to determine whether mass spectrometry imaging could assist in the diagnosis and risk stratification of atypical Spitzoid neoplasms.[11]

In 2009, we founded the International Spitzoid Neoplasm Study Group. The mission statement of the group is to (1) establish cooperation among dermatopathologists throughout the world in order to research Spitzoid lesions; (2) share information and case material so that each participant benefits using a large database; and (3) allow all contributors to be rewarded by participation in publications. Members of the International Spitzoid Neoplasm Study Group together with other collaborators provided more than 200 cases of atypical Spitzoid neoplasms for a retrospective study, which involved centers from 11 countries and 11 US institutions.[11]

We performed mass spectrometry imaging in a large series of patients atypical Spitzoid neoplasms and available clinical follow-up. In each case we compared the diagnosis rendered by mass spectrometry imaging with the histopathologic diagnosis and also correlated the diagnoses with clinical outcomes. Patients were divided into 4 clinical groups representing best to worst clinical behavior. The association among mass spectrometry imaging findings, histopathologic diagnoses, and clinical groups was assessed.

When analyzing atypical Spitzoid neoplasms for which neither melanoma nor nevus was favored histopathologically, mass spectrometry imaging seemed to be more accurate in predicting the benign character of atypical Spitzoid neoplasms than histopathology and correlated better with their clinical behavior (**Fig. 3**). Histopathology had a tendency to overdiagnose either atypical features or malignancy. A strong association was found between the diagnosis of Spitzoid melanoma by mass spectrometry imaging and an adverse clinical outcome when clinical group 1 (no recurrence or metastasis beyond a sentinel node) was compared with groups 2, 3, and 4 (recurrence of disease, metastases or death). In addition, the diagnosis of Spitzoid melanoma by mass spectrometry imaging was statistically strongly associated with adverse clinical behavior. Mass spectrometry imaging analysis using a proteomic signature may be able to provide more reliable diagnosis and clinically useful and statistically significant risk assessment of

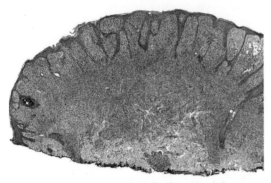

Fig. 3. A dome-shaped and asymmetric proliferation of large epithelioid melanocytes in sheets. This patient was a 15-year-old girl with a lesion on the neck. A histopathologic diagnosis of atypical Spitzoid neoplasm. Because Spitzoid melanoma could not be excluded, in addition to wide excision, the patient underwent sentinel lymph node dissection and had negative nodes. Mass spectrometry imaging rendered a diagnosis of Spitz nevus. The patient is alive and with no evidence of disease at 4 years of follow-up.

atypical Spitzoid neoplasms, beyond the information provided by histology and other ancillary techniques.

### Metastasis versus benign nevus
The distinction between a metastasis and a nevus is sometimes difficult to make, but it is very important for determining the patient's clinical staging and management. Here is an example of a case in which mass spectrometry imaging was very helpful.[12] A 37-year-old pregnant woman was diagnosed with a 2.2-mm-thick melanoma on the right upper arm in her late pregnancy. Ulceration was absent;

there were 25 mitoses/mm$^2$, and intravascular invasion was present. The patient had a term delivery by a cesarean section, at which time a wide excision and lymph node dissection were undertaken. The newborn baby had several atypical melanocytic lesions on the back and flank (Fig. 4). It was of paramount importance to determine whether these were congenital nevi or metastases from the mother's melanoma. In the latter case, the mother's clinical stage had to be upgraded to stage IV.

Biopsies from 2 of the baby's atypical melanocytic lesions were sent for histopathologic examination. In the mother's melanoma, there was a nodular area composed of small melanocytes with high nuclear to cytoplasmic ratio. The melanocytes within the 2 biopsied lesions from the baby resembled the melanocytes from the nodular portion of the mother's melanoma. Because of the histologic similarities, it was difficult to make a definitive diagnosis of either benign nevi or melanoma metastases from the mother's malignant melanoma. The mother's melanoma and the baby's 2 melanocytic lesions, were subjected to mass spectrometry imaging analysis and compared (Fig. 5). The baby's lesions were classified by mass spectrometry as nevi and had a different proteomic profile than the mother's melanoma (Fig. 6).

### Proliferative nodules in congenital melanocytic nevi versus developing melanoma
Another difficult area in dermatopathology is the distinction between a proliferative nodule and malignant melanoma arising in the background of a congenital melanocytic nevus. Both can present with large, pleomorphic, and atypical melanocytes, with prominent nucleoli and numerous

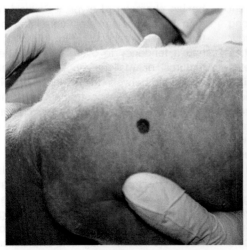
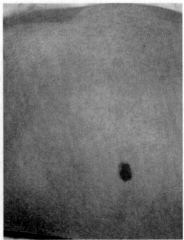

Fig. 4. Two atypical melanocytic lesions in a newborn baby from the back (*left*) and right flank (*right*).

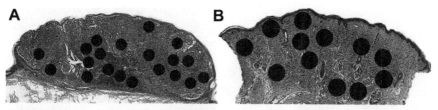

Fig. 5. The melanoma of the mother (*A*) and one of the atypical melanocytic lesions from the baby (*B*) with marked areas to be studied by mass spectrometry imaging.

mitotic figures. In some cases, large areas of congenital melanocytic nevi are proliferative and closely mimic melanoma.

Mass spectrometry imaging can be used in cases in which it may be difficult histopathologically to make a diagnosis of either a proliferative nodule within a congenital melanocytic nevus or melanoma developing in the setting of a congenital nevus. We can illustrate that with a consultation case we received from an otherwise healthy Chinese baby who was born with a large, approximately 4.5 cm in diameter, melanocytic lesion on the scalp.[13] In 2 months, the lesion doubled its size to approximately 10 cm in diameter and was focally ulcerated and necrotic (**Fig.** 7A). An excision of the entire lesion with 1-cm margin followed by a full-thickness skin graft was performed. A diagnosis of malignant melanoma was rendered by pathologists at 2 Chinese hospitals (**Fig.** 8). The surgeon who performed the operation and followed up the patient believed that this was a benign lesion and not melanoma, based on the clinical behavior. He requested our opinion and we offered, in addition to histopathologic examination, to analyze the lesion by mass spectrometry imaging, which classified it as benign nevus. The diagnosis of benign nevus better correlates with the clinical outcome; the child is alive and free of disease 4 years after the surgery (see **Fig.** 7B).

### Challenging melanocytic lesions

Mass spectrometry imaging may be helpful in the analysis of challenging melanocytic lesions of different types. We studied large numbers of different types of melanoma and compared them with banal melanocytic nevi.[14] After a molecular signature was established, we applied this signature in the analysis and diagnosis of challenging melanocytic lesions. In a case of a

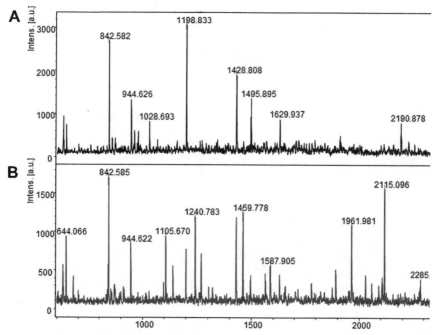

Fig. 6. The proteomic composition of the mother's melanoma (*A*) and one of the baby's atypical melanocytic lesion (*B*) is different . Intens. [a.u.], Intensity in arbitrary units.

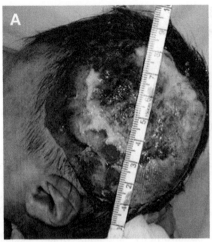
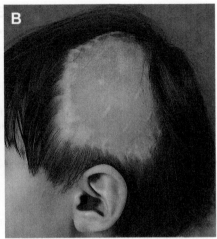

Fig. 7. (*A*) Large protruding mass with foci of ulceration and necrosis on the scalp of the baby at 2 months of age. (*B*) A full-thickness skin graft on the left scalp of the child at 2.5 years of age.

50-year-old woman with a new lesion on the left thigh there were compelling histopathologic features in favor of malignant melanoma and a diagnosis of melanoma with a tumor thickness of 4.75 mm and 1 mitosis/mm$^2$ was rendered (**Fig. 9**).

Subsequently, the patient underwent sentinel lymph node dissection and had 1 positive sentinel lymph node. This case was included in our study as Spitzoid melanoma. Mass spectrometry imaging analysis diagnosed the lesion as benign. A repeated analysis provided the same diagnosis. Additional molecular studies were performed and no copy number or any other abnormalities were detected. The patient is alive and with no evidence of disease 7 years after the initial diagnosis.

This case illustrates well the ability of mass spectrometry imaging to help in the diagnosis of challenging melanocytic lesions and their stratification and risk analysis. This method can provide biological insight that is not attainable by standard histology, examining the molecular composition of tumors, and delivering an objective diagnosis based on proteomic differences, as well as bringing insight about disease outcome and treatment response.

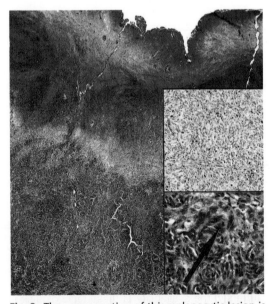

Fig. 8. The upper portion of this melanocytic lesion is completely necrotic. Underneath is a dense proliferation of melanocytes in back-to-back nests. The upper inset shows high proliferative activity. Many nuclei label with ki-67. The arrow points to a mitotic figure in the lower inset.

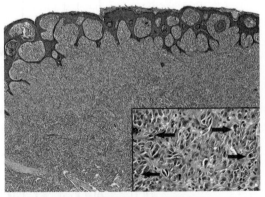

Fig. 9. A predominantly dermal proliferation of melanocytes organized in confluent nests and in sheets. The melanocytes do not mature with their descent into the dermis. Numerous mitotic figures are seen in the inset (*arrows*).

## SUMMARY

Mass spectrometry can be a useful tool for the diagnosis of skin cancer. Mass spectrometry imaging is able to identify unique molecular signatures to aid in the diagnosis, particularly of challenging melanocytic lesions. The incorporation of a proteomic signature may improve the diagnosis, prediction of outcomes, and risk stratification for patients with atypical Spitzoid neoplasms and other types of challenging melanocytic lesions.

## REFERENCES

1. Miteva M, Lazova R. Spitz nevus and atypical spitzoid neoplasm. Semin Cutan Med Surg 2010;29(3): 165–73.
2. Farmer ER, Gonin R, Hanna MP. Discordance in the histopathologic diagnosis of melanoma and melanocytic nevi between expert pathologists. Hum Pathol 1996;27(6):528–31.
3. Ackerman AB. Discordance among expert pathologists in diagnosis of melanocytic neoplasms. Hum Pathol 1996;27(11):1115–6.
4. Barnhill RL, Argenyi ZB, From L, et al. Atypical Spitz nevi/tumors: lack of consensus for diagnosis, discrimination from melanoma, and prediction of outcome. Hum Pathol 1999;30(5):513–20.
5. Cerroni L, Barnhill R, Elder D, et al. Melanocytic tumors of uncertain malignant potential: results of a tutorial held at the XXIX Symposium of the International Society of Dermatopathology in Graz, October 2008. Am J Surg Pathol 2010;34(3):314–26.
6. Yanagisawa K, Shyr Y, Xu BJ, et al. Proteomic patterns of tumour subsets in non-small-cell lung cancer. Lancet 2003;362(9382):433–9.
7. Cornett DS, Mobley JA, Dias EC, et al. A novel histology-directed strategy for MALDI-MS tissue profiling that improves throughput and cellular specificity in human breast cancer. Mol Cell Proteomics 2006;5(10):1975–83.
8. Conrad DH, Goyette J, Thomas PS. Proteomics as a method for early detection of cancer: a review of proteomics, exhaled breath condensate, and lung cancer screening. J Gen Intern Med 2008; 23(Suppl 1):78–84.
9. Nimesh S, Mohottalage S, Vincent R, et al. Current status and future perspectives of mass spectrometry imaging. Int J Mol Sci 2013;14(6): 11277–301.
10. Lazova R, Seeley EH, Keenan M, et al. Imaging mass spectrometry–a new and promising method to differentiate Spitz nevi from spitzoid malignant melanomas. Am J Dermatopathol 2012;34(1): 82–90.
11. Lazova R, Seeley EH, Kutzner H, et al. Imaging mass spectrometry assists in the classification of diagnostically challenging atypical spitzoid neoplasms. J Am Acad Dermatol 2016;75(6): 1176–86.e4.
12. Alomari AK, Glusac EJ, Choi J, et al. Congenital nevi versus metastatic melanoma in a newborn to a mother with malignant melanoma - diagnosis supported by sex chromosome analysis and imaging mass spectrometry. J Cutan Pathol 2015;42(10): 757–64.
13. Lazova R, Yang Z, El Habr C, et al. Mass Spectrometry Imaging Can Distinguish on a Proteomic Level Between Proliferative Nodules Within a Benign Congenital Nevus and Malignant Melanoma. Am J Dermatopathol 2017. [Epub ahead of print].
14. Lazova R, Seeley HE. Mass Spectrometry Imaging – an objective and reliable method to differentiate between benign melanocytic nevi and malignant melanomas. J Cut Pathol 2016;43:e74.

# Assessing Skin Cancer Using Epidermal Genetic Information Retrieved by Adhesive Patch Skin Surface Sampling

Nayoung Lee, MD[a], Alon Scope, MD[b], Harold Rabinovitz, MD[a,c],*

## KEYWORDS

- Epidermal genetic information retrieval • Melanoma • Nevi • Noninvasive • Diagnosis

## KEY POINTS

- Epidermal genetic information retrieval (EGIR) is a noninvasive diagnostic method involving the application of adhesive tape onto the skin's surface to recover genomic material from the epidermis.
- Preliminary studies have shown the potential of this technology to aid clinicians in differentiating between melanomas and nevi.
- Although not meant to replace a biopsy, EGIR by adhesive patch sampling can guide the decision on surgical biopsy in patients who may have numerous nevi or in those with a suspect lesion on a cosmetically sensitive area.

## INTRODUCTION

It is widely accepted that the early detection of melanoma improves survival.[1] In order to properly evaluate a lesion concerning for melanoma, an excisional biopsy is typically performed. For some patients, such as those with a questionable lesion in a cosmetically sensitive area or patients with numerous atypical melanocytic nevi, the risk of morbidity associated with such a procedure should be carefully weighed against the likelihood that the lesion in question is malignant. Although dermoscopy has improved the accuracy of melanoma diagnosis, its utility is highly user dependent; even for pigmented lesions specialists, the number of benign lesions biopsied for every melanoma detected ranges from 5 to 1 at best to 15 to 1.[2]

Advances in technology have led to improved noninvasive diagnostic modalities for melanoma.[3–12] However, for many of these approaches, advanced training is required and application is user dependent. A more objective noninvasive test with high sensitivity and specificity that could minimize interuser variability would be highly beneficial for improving diagnosis of melanoma and for reducing the number of unnecessary skin biopsies.

In recent years, a new method was introduced as an alternative to the aforementioned technologies. Adhesive patch skin surface sampling, also

Disclosures: The authors have no financial disclosures or conflicts of interest.
[a] Department of Dermatology and Cutaneous Surgery, University of Miami Miller School of Medicine, 1600 NW 10th Avenue, Miami, FL 33136, USA; [b] Department of Dermatology, Sheba Medical Center, Sackler School of Medicine, Tel Aviv University, Tel Hashomer 5262000, Israel; [c] Private Practice, Skin and Cancer Associates, Plantation, FL 33324, USA
* Corresponding author. Private Practice, Skin and Cancer Associates, Plantation, FL 33324.
*E-mail address:* harold@admcorp.com

Dermatol Clin 35 (2017) 521–524
http://dx.doi.org/10.1016/j.det.2017.06.013

known as epidermal genetic information retrieval (EGIR) (DermTech International, Inc, La Jolla, CA) is distinct in its analysis of genomic material from the lesion in question using noninvasive methods. EGIR is the focus of the present article.

## EPIDERMAL GENETIC INFORMATION RETRIEVAL

EGIR involves obtaining and analyzing RNA from epidermal cells for the expression of genes associated with melanoma. The exact mechanism of how RNA originating from melanocytes is found in the superficial epidermis and is thus detected by EGIR is not yet known. Some investigators hypothesize that this may be because of shedding of melanocytes toward the superficial epidermis, or pagetoid spread of melanocytes, or exchange of subcellular material between the melanocytes and keratinocytes.[13]

EGIR was first developed for the study of other dermatologic conditions.[14] It has been used to differentiate allergic from irritant contact dermatitis and to analyze the expression of specific cytokines in psoriatic plaques by quantitative reverse transcription polymerase chain reaction (RT-PCR) assay.[15] Wong and colleagues[14] later found that RNA obtained via adhesive patch sampling was suitable for use in DNA microarray experiments and that it relayed information from epidermal cells located below the stratum corneum. This finding was the basis for adhesive patch sampling of melanocytic lesions for a diagnostic purpose. In order to investigate whether the adhesive patch sampling could distinguish a melanoma from a nevus, an adhesive tape was applied to the surface of the lesion to retrieve epidermal cells, from which RNA

was extracted using RT-PCR. This RNA was then hybridized to a DNA microarray chip consisting of numerous genes to determine the gene expression profile of the lesion.

The preliminary investigation by Wachsman and colleagues[16] was designed to compare the gene expression profiles of melanoma and benign nevi. The investigators performed EGIR by applying 4 adhesive tape disks onto pigmented lesions (**Fig. 1**), followed by surgical removal of the lesions for histopathologic analysis by 2 independent dermatopathologists. In total, 20 melanomas (9 in situ and 11 invasive), 62 nevi, and 17 nonlesional normal skin samples were included in the study. Lesions suspicious for melanoma that were bleeding or ulcerated were excluded. RNA from the 4 disks was pooled and amplified using quantitative RT-PCR and profiled for gene expression on a gene chip containing 47,000 transcripts. By this method, differential expression levels among melanomas, nevi, and normal skin of 317 genes were identified; of these, 89 genes were shown to be differentially expressed between melanomas and nevi. These results showed that EGIR has potential for being used to distinguish melanomas from nevi.

In 2011, Wachsman and colleagues[17] showed that EGIR performed on 202 melanocytic lesions identified 312 genes that were differentially expressed among melanomas, nevi, and normal human skin. On subsequent EGIR testing of biopsy-confirmed melanocytic neoplasms, including 37 melanomas and 37 nevi, these 312 candidate genes were further narrowed down to 17 genes that were able to differentiate melanomas from nevi with a reported sensitivity of 100% and specificity of 88%.[17] These 17 genes included genes involved in cell

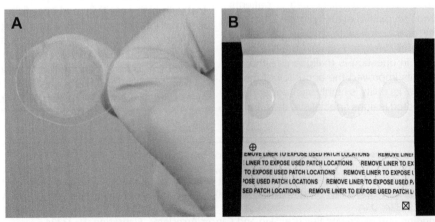

**Fig. 1.** EGIR. (*A*) An adhesive tape disk allows retrieval of epidermal cells. (*B*) Four adhesive patch disks are successively applied to and removed from each lesion. RNA from the 4 disks is pooled and amplified using quantitative RT-PCR and profiled for gene expression. (*Courtesy of* DermTech, La Jolla, CA; with permission.)

death, cellular development, hair and skin development, and neurologic disease.[17] Using this 17-gene classifier for melanoma, the investigators were able to classify correctly 10 out of 10 specimens of lentigo maligna as melanoma. Of 35 benign lesions, 22 solar lentigines were correctly classified as benign. The other 13 lesions tested positive for melanoma by EGIR, but were diagnosed by histopathology as benign; however, on repeat sectioning and reviewing, 1 of these 13 lesions contained a focus of invasive melanoma. Again, this study showed the potential of EGIR for discerning melanoma from nevi and the future possibility for being used in the clinic for noninvasive testing of melanocytic neoplasms.

In another study designed to develop an in vitro diagnostic assay for clinical detection of melanoma, 91 lesions were assessed by adhesive patch sampling and quantitative RT-PCR for expression of pairwise combinations of genes from a previously established 15-gene classifier. The lesions were then submitted for histopathologic diagnosis by 3 blinded dermatopathologists. The gene pair consisting of c-maf-inducing protein (CMIP) and long intergenic non-protein coding RNA 518 (LINC00518) showed the best results in discriminating melanomas from benign lesions. The results were further validated in a set of 64 lesions consisting of 42 melanomas and 22 nevi. CMIP, a gene involved in downregulating nuclear factor kappa B (NF-kB), thereby promoting apoptosis, was found to be downregulated in melanomas compared with nevi. It was postulated that CMIP may be implicated in melanomagenesis.

In contrast, LINC00518 messenger RNA was upregulated in melanoma compared with nevi. LINC00518 encodes a regulatory RNA belonging to a group of long noncoding RNAs; although these RNAs do not code for proteins, they were found to colocalize with a genomic region that frequent displays, in melanomas, gains in the gene copy number. These long noncoding RNAs have been shown to play a role in cell proliferation and differentiation. Gerami and colleagues[18] showed that the expression levels of these 2 genes, CMIP and LINC00518, were able to differentiate melanomas from nevi with a sensitivity of 97.6% and a specificity of 72.7%. Unlike the previously mentioned initial studies using the adhesive patch sampling technique to assess melanocytic lesions, in this study, gene expression levels were ascertained using quantitative RT-PCR without the use of DNA microarrays. By replacing the microarray with a more cost-effective and more rapid diagnostic tool, this study made EGIR a more applicable test for clinical use.

Similar to the earlier studies by Wachsman and colleagues,[16,17] 6 of the histopathologically diagnosed nevi showed gene expression–based scores consistent with melanoma. Out of these 6 cases, 3 were diagnosed as dysplastic nevus with severe atypia; thus, Gerami and colleagues[18] conjectured that it was unclear whether the results for these 6 lesions were gene expression false-positives or very early melanomas that defied morphologic recognition via histopathology.

The aforementioned studies have led to the development of the Pigmented Lesion Assay, which tests for the expression of 2 genes that have been shown to be expressed at higher levels in melanoma: LINC00518 and Preferentially Expressed Antigen in Melanoma (PRAME). If expression in either of these 2 genes is detected, an additional set of genes that are differentially expressed in melanoma and nevi, including CMIP, are tested to calculate a numerical score that assesses the risk that the lesion is a melanoma.

In a recent validation study by Gerami and colleagues[19] that examined 398 biopsied lesions, including 87 melanomas and 311 nonmelanomas consisting of mostly benign melanocytic proliferations and some nonmelanocytic lesions, such as seborrheic keratosis and basal cell carcinomas, this 2-gene signature detected melanomas with a sensitivity of 91% and a specificity of 69%. Although in the near future this test is not meant to replace a diagnostic biopsy, it has potential for serving as an adjunct to the clinical decision of whether to biopsy an equivocal melanocytic lesion.

## SUMMARY

EGIR by adhesive patch sampling has potential for assisting in the bedside diagnosis of melanoma, especially in patients with numerous clinically atypical nevi or those with a concerning pigmented lesion on a cosmetically sensitive area. In conjunction with the physician's clinical judgment and evaluation using imaging devices, such as dermoscopy and confocal microscopy, EGIR can help guide physicians in the decision to perform an excisional biopsy.

Further research is needed, such as large pivotal studies in the clinical setting, and testing whether EGIR could be used on amelanotic melanomas, acral lentiginous melanomas, and mucosal melanomas. Another interesting area of study could be whether gene expression of melanomas varies by melanoma thickness or biological behavior, in a way that could make EGIR useful for prognostic purposes. In addition,

EGIR has the potential to identify future biomarkers that would be helpful in tailoring targeted therapy for individual patients with melanoma.

## REFERENCES

1. Balch CM, Gershenwald JE, Soong SJ, et al. Final version of 2009 AJCC melanoma staging and classification. J Clin Oncol 2009;27(36):6199–206.
2. Wilson RL, Yentzer BA, Isom SP, et al. How good are US dermatologists at discriminating skin cancers? A number-needed-to-treat analysis. J Dermatolog Treat 2012;23(1):65–9.
3. Stevenson AD, Mickan S, Mallett S, et al. Systematic review of diagnostic accuracy of reflectance confocal microscopy for melanoma diagnosis in patients with clinically equivocal skin lesions. Dermatol Pract Concept 2013;3(4):19–27.
4. Alarcon I, Carrera C, Palou J, et al. Impact of in vivo reflectance confocal microscopy on the number needed to treat melanoma in doubtful lesions. Br J Dermatol 2014;170(4):802–8.
5. Pellacani G, Pepe P, Casari A, et al. Reflectance confocal microscopy as a second-level examination in skin oncology improves diagnostic accuracy and saves unnecessary excisions: a longitudinal prospective study. Br J Dermatol 2014;171(5):1044–51.
6. Glud M, Gniadecki R, Drzewiecki KT. Spectrophotometric intracutaneous analysis versus dermoscopy for the diagnosis of pigmented skin lesions: prospective, double-blind study in a secondary reference centre. Melanoma Res 2009;19(3):176–9.
7. Haniffa MA, Lloyd JJ, Lawrence CM. The use of a spectrophotometric intracutaneous analysis device in the real-time diagnosis of melanoma in the setting of a melanoma screening clinic. Br J Dermatol 2007; 156(6):1350–2.
8. Monheit G, Cognetta AB, Ferris L, et al. The performance of MelaFind: a prospective multicenter study. Arch Dermatol 2011;147(2):188–94.
9. Rigel DS, Roy M, Yoo J, et al. Impact of guidance from a computer-aided multispectral digital skin lesion analysis device on decision to biopsy lesions clinically suggestive of melanoma. Arch Dermatol 2012;148(4):541–3.
10. Hauschild A, Chen SC, Weichenthal M, et al. To excise or not: impact of MelaFind on German dermatologists' decisions to biopsy atypical lesions. J Dtsch Dermatol Ges 2014;12(7):606–14.
11. Mohr P, Birgersson U, Berking C, et al. Electrical impedance spectroscopy as a potential adjunct diagnostic tool for cutaneous melanoma. Skin Res Technol 2013;19(2):75–83.
12. Malvehy J, Hauschild A, Curiel-Lewandrowski C, et al. Clinical performance of the Nevisense system in cutaneous melanoma detection: an international, multicentre, prospective and blinded clinical trial on efficacy and safety. Br J Dermatol 2014;171(5):1099–107.
13. Wachsman W. Clinical genomics for melanoma detection. In: Rigell DS, editor. Cancer of the skin. London: Elsevier; 2011. p. 429–33.
14. Wong R, Tran V, Morhenn V, et al. Use of RT-PCR and DNA microarrays to characterize RNA recovered by non-invasive tape harvesting of normal and inflamed skin. J Invest Dermatol 2004;123(1):159–67.
15. Benson NR, Papenfuss J, Wong R, et al. An analysis of select pathogenic messages in lesional and non-lesional psoriatic skin using non-invasive tape harvesting. J Invest Dermatol 2006;126(10):2234–41.
16. Wachsman W, Zapala M, Udall D, et al. Differentiation of melanoma from dysplastic nevi in suspicious pigmented skin lesions by non-invasive tape stripping. J Invest Dermatol 2007;127:S145.
17. Wachsman W, Morhenn V, Palmer T, et al. Noninvasive genomic detection of melanoma. Br J Dermatol 2011;164(4):797–806.
18. Gerami P, Alsobrook JP 2nd, Palmer TJ, et al. Development of a novel noninvasive adhesive patch test for the evaluation of pigmented lesions of the skin. J Am Acad Dermatol 2014;71(2):237–44.
19. Gerami P, Yao Z, Polsky D, et al. Development and validation of a noninvasive 2-gene molecular assay for cutaneous melanoma. J Am Acad Dermatol 2017;76(1):114–20.e2.

# Detection of Genetic Aberrations in the Assessment and Prognosis of Melanoma

Whitney A. High, MD, JD, MEng*

## KEYWORDS

- Atypical nevus • Atypical Spitz nevus • Comparative genetic hybridization • Diagnosis
- Gene expression profiling • Fluorescent in situ hybridization • Melanoma • Prognosis

## KEY POINTS

- Melanoma is an often subjective diagnosis made using light microscopy and H&E staining, and the dermatopathologic impression may be augmented by other means.
- Additional means for augmenting a histologic impression of melanoma include immunohistochemical (IHC) staining and/or genetic testing.
- In problematic lesions, IHC stains used to refine or refute the diagnosis of melanoma may include Melan-A/MART-1, S100, Ki67, p16, and HMB-45.
- In problematic lesions, adjunctive genetic assessment of melanoma used to refine or refute the diagnosis of melanoma include comparative genetic hybridization (CGH), fluorescent in situ hybridization (FISH), and gene expression profiling (GEP).
- There exist new genetic means to stratify risk and gauge prognosis in melanoma, and as additional adjunctive therapy expands, and surveillance protocols are further refined, growth in this area is anticipated.

## INTRODUCTION

At present, the histologic diagnosis of skin cancer remains a critical step in the evaluation and management of skin disease. For the foreseeable future, and from a medicolegal standpoint in particular, a histologic report of cancer is requisite for additional intervention. For example, melanoma requires histologic staging information (eg, Breslow depth, presence/absence of ulceration, dermal mitotic activity) to select appropriate management. Even entrance into oncologic trials for melanoma, using new agents and new protocols, is affected by this histologic staging information.

In dermatopathology, the underlying practical means for rendering a cancer diagnosis has changed little in the last 140 years.[1] Each work day, dermatopathologists in the United States rely heavily on hematoxylin and eosin (H&E) staining and standard light microscopy to render most diagnoses. Moreover, even when a diagnosis is augmented by an adjunctive technique of some sort, H&E evaluation still remains a cornerstone or "back-bone" of the diagnostic schema.

Yet, reliance on simple histomorphologic assessment of tumors (ie, the physical appearance and arrangement of cancerous cells under the microscope) to predict genetic potential (ie,

University of Colorado School of Medicine, 12605 E 16th Avenue, Aurora, CO 80045, USA
* 12635 East Montview Boulevard, Suite 160, Aurora, CO 80045.
E-mail address: Whitney.High@ucdenver.edu

Dermatol Clin 35 (2017) 525–536
http://dx.doi.org/10.1016/j.det.2017.06.015
0733-8635/17/© 2017 Elsevier Inc. All rights reserved.

derm.theclinics.com

possession of genetic characteristics to become fatal metastatic disease) is not without consequence. Parenthetically, in the social sciences, reliance on outward appearances to predict behavior is considered an inefficient means of analysis (ie, so-called profiling)[2]; yet in dermatopathology, variations on this same type of pattern recognition are ubiquitously used.

In truth, particularly with regard to melanocytic neoplasia, there remain fundamental disagreements, even among dermatopathology experts, as to what represents melanoma.[3–7] Additionally, it has been demonstrated, repeatedly, that with regard to the histomorphologic assessment of melanoma, discrepancies among key histologic features exist.[7,8] It has been estimated by some experts that about 10% of pigmented lesions examined at expert tertiary melanoma centers may defy a singular confident diagnosis.[4]

Therefore, if specialty care providers in dermatology and dermatopathology desire to know what a skin neoplasm is capable of doing, at least in terms of yielding metastatic disease and patient demise, it is imperative that they develop and adopt means of genetic assessment, for it is precisely such genetic potential that is of concern in caring for patients.

This article focuses on available techniques used for the evaluation of melanocytic neoplasms. The reason for this focus is practical in nature: this is where the bulk of available adjunctive genetic techniques currently lie. At present, there are not significant and useful genetic techniques, in widespread use, for the evaluation of basal cell carcinoma or squamous cell carcinoma, although there is some interest in the latter. The evaluation of dermatofibrosarcoma protuberans, by means of a break-apart fluorescent in situ hybridization (FISH) probe that identifies a specific translocation, permeates clinical practice, yet this tumor is relatively rare.

Although cutaneous lymphoma may be the subject of genetic studies to demonstrate clonality, again as an adjunctive measure to light microscopy and immunohistochemistry (IHC) studies, clonality is not the equivalent of malignancy, nor is the absence of a detected clone exclusive of malignancy. Hence, given its lesser utility, and the fact this is a largely subspecialty concern, such a discussion is better reserved for an exclusive discourse on lymphoproliferative disorders.

## DIAGNOSTIC MELANOMA ASSESSMENT
### Lack of a Gold Standard

The assessment of melanoma is sometimes highly subjective. There are disagreements, even among experts, as to which challenging melanocytic neoplasms represent atypical/dysplastic/Clark nevi or melanoma, or which challenging spitzoid lesions represent classic Spitz nevi or atypical Spitz nevi/tumors or spitzoid melanoma. Complicating matters is that there is no singular gold standard, short of actual biologic behavior over time, which can prove something is, or is not, melanoma.

Moreover, where a tertiary care facility has overturned an assessment of melanoma rendered by an outside facility, or in the alternative, where a tertiary facility has rendered an assessment of melanoma, where an outside facility had not, there is bias to assume this second opinion is correct. Although perhaps a reasonable first assumption, given the expertise and depth of experience at a tertiary facility, in the absence of an adverse outcome experienced by the patient, there is no way to guarantee a second opinion is any more, or any less, correct than the first opinion rendered.

What if a person had melanoma, but it was treated as a severely atypical nevus, and the person simply survived? What if a person had a severely atypical nevus, but received treatment of melanoma that was unnecessary, but difficult to separate from melanoma survival?

In sum, the lack of a definitive gold standard, except in cases where an adverse outcome is experienced by the patient, poses a challenge to investigations of genetic diagnostic techniques[9]; this fact must be kept in mind in all of the discourse to follow.

### Immunohistochemical Stains

Although the realm of H&E staining and light microscopy has changed little in the last century, the development and addition of IHC stains is a more recent development. The groundwork for modern IHC techniques was laid in the 1940s through 1960s, and widespread use of IHC began in earnest in the late 1980s.[10]

In brief, IHC represents a means to detect specific antigens in or on cells based on an antigen-antibody reaction that is recognized at the light microscopic level because of final application of a material that produces a visible color. Antigen retrieval is performed, and then a primary monoclonal antibody is applied. This antibody is directed against a specific tissue antigen. A secondary antibody is then applied that localizes to the first antibody. Conjugated to this secondary antibody are molecules of either horseradish peroxidase enzyme or alkaline phosphatase enzyme. Finally, a chromagen is applied that reacts with the conjugated enzyme to yield brown or red pigment deposition that is visualized under the microscope. The existence of both brown and red chromagen systems mean that under certain conditions two antibodies may be tested at the same time, yielding two different colors (discussed later).

## No Single Melanoma Marker Exists

There are several IHC stains are useful for studying melanocytic lesions, but it is import to stress bluntly that no single melanoma marker exists by IHC. Although some IHC markers are useful in suggesting a melanocytic process is benign or malignant, this is merely adjunctive information that must be interpreted in the context of all available data, including assessment by H&E staining alone. Certain patterns of IHC staining, although sometimes suggestive of melanoma, may at other times simply be spurious and inconsequential.

IHC markers are only adjunctive tools that must be placed in context, and do not necessarily supersede traditional morphologic clues provided by light microscopy, to include asymmetry, pagetoid scatter, nuclear pleomorphism, hyperchromasia, irregular nuclear contour, irregular nesting of melanocytes, poor maturation in the dermis, and dermal mitotic activity.

## Immunohistiochemical Stains Useful for Diagnosis of Melanoma

The following IHC markers are often used in the evaluation of pigmented lesions and the characteristics of each is discussed next.

### S100

A sensitive marker for melanocytic neoplasms, with about 95% of primary cutaneous melanomas expressing this antibody.[11–14] Desmoplastic/spindle cell melanoma often expresses S100, even though these types of melanoma are typically negative for melan-A/MART-1 and HMB-45. However, S100 expression is not specific for only melanoma, and S100 is also expressed by normal melanocytes, nervous tissue, myoepithelial cells, adipocytes, chondrocytes, and Langerhans cells.[11]

### Melan-A/MART-1

Benign and malignant melanocytes express the Melan A/MART-1 antigen, which is detected by the A103 and M2-7C10 clonal antibodies, respectively.[15–17] In practical clinical parlance the terms are interchangeable. Although a sensitive and specific marker for melanocytes, it is important to recognize that desmoplastic/spindle cell melanoma is consistently negative for Melan A/MART-1 antibodies. Lastly, Melan A/MART-1 can yield a confusing pattern of staining called "pseudonesting," where the immunostain marks a disputed mixture of inflammatory cells, melanocytes, and keratinocytes at the dermoepidermal junction that can lead to erroneous impressions of melanoma in situ.[18,19]

### Ki-67/MIB-1

Ki-67/MIB-1 is a proliferation marker used to identify cells that are progressing through the cell cycle and preparing for mitosis. In one study, common and dysplastic nevi showed about 1% of melanocyte nuclei to mark (most often near the dermoepidermal junction or in the superficial dermis), whereas in melanoma, about 16.4% of melanocyte nuclei marked, particularly in the deeper extents. This and other investigations led to a postulated "rule of thumb" for difficult pigmented lesions where benignity is favored by a low Ki67/MIB-1 proliferative index of less than 2%, whereas malignancy is favored by a Ki67/MIB-1 higher proliferative index of greater than 10%, with indeterminate lesions occupying a middle ground.[20,21]

Moreover, Melan A/MART-1 IHC staining, using a red chromagen, may be combined with Ki67 IHC staining, using a brown chromagen, to yield a "double stain" (KiMart) that may be used to assess the proliferative index of melanocytes, with lesser confounding by other cell types (see case study 1).

### HMB-45

HMB-45 is an antibody directed at the gp100 protein of melanocytes. In benign acquired nevi HMB-45 expression is often limited to melanocytes at dermoepidermal junctional and in the papillary dermis, with lesser marking in the deeper dermis.[22] This pattern reinforces the normal maturation of nevi, and it is referred to as "zonation." Lack of zonation with HMB-45 is a concerning finding in some situations; however, melanocytic neoplasms with dusty cytoplasm, such as clonal nevi or deep penetrating nevi, represent important exceptions and do not "zone" with HMB-45, but this is not evidence of malignancy per se.

### p16

p16 is a tumor-suppressor protein encoded on chromosome 9. Most benign nevi manifest a mosaic pattern of p16 expression, with more than 25% of cells marking with either nuclear or cytoplasmic expression. In one study examining p16 expression among 46 atypical Spitz tumors and 42 melanoma specimens, decreased nuclear expression of p16 was three-fold more likely in melanoma than in Spitz tumors ($P = .004$), and loss of both nuclear and cytoplasmic dermal p16 expression was eight-fold more likely in melanoma ($P = .01$).[23] In another study of p16 staining, using 15 desmoplastic Spitz nevi and 11 desmoplastic melanomas, all cases of Spitz nevi showed p16 expression, whereas 81.2% of desmoplastic melanomas were p16 negative, and 18.8% of melanomas were only weakly p16 positive.[24] It is important to stress that loss of p16 expression is not simply an immediate marker of melanoma, but loss of p16 expression could indicate biallelic loss of chromosome 9p21, which in turn, is an adverse prognostic marker in spitzoid neoplasia. Particularly in the realm of spitzoid neoplasia, lesions with lost p16 expression by IHC should be treated with greater suspicion than those that express p16 in a normal fashion.[25]

### Case study 1

A 14-year-old boy presented with a dark-brown, pedunculated lesion on the flank that had been growing over the last 4 months. The lesion was sampled, and despite his relative youth, the results of H&E/light microscopy and IHC staining were interpreted as melanoma (**Fig. 1**). This diagnosis was subsequently reviewed at a second academic institution and there was full concurrence in the diagnosis of melanoma.

## USE OF GENETIC TESTING IN MELANOMA

Current widely available genetic testing modalities to augment a diagnostic impression formed by H&E/light microscopy are divided into three classes: (1) comparative genomic hybridization (CGH), (2) FISH, and (3) gene expression profiling (GEP).

### Comparative Genomic Hybridization

CGH is a technique that detects genome-wide changes in DNA copy number, but it does not detect actual mutations.[26,27] Current microarray-based methods of CGH allow for maximum resolution, and can even detect single copy number changes.[28] Use of chromosomal analysis in the diagnosis of melanocytic lesions is premised on a concept that genomic aberrations are common

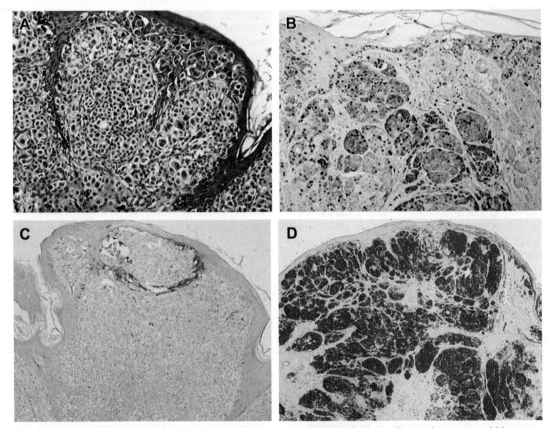

**Fig. 1.** On histologic examination, this pedunculated pigmented lesion from the flank of a 14-year-old boy manifested (*A*) markedly atypical epithelioid cells, with pagetoid extent, dermal mitotic activity, and no dermal maturation (H&E, original magnification ×400); (*B*) an aberrant and elevated proliferative index by KiMart IHC staining (MART-1 [*red*], Ki67 [*brown*], original magnification ×200); (*C*) complete loss of any P16 expression among melanocytes (original magnification ×100); and (*D*) aberrant retention of HMB-45 in the deep dermal nests (original magnification ×40).

in melanoma, but generally absent in benign nevi, with most melanomas possessing an average of greater than five genomic aberrations.[27] Common genetic anomalies found in melanoma include gains in chromosomes 6p, 1q, 7p, 7q, 8q, 17q, and 20q, and/or losses of 9p, 9q, 10q, 10p, 6q, and 11q.[28] Spitz nevi often demonstrate isolated gains of 11p or 7q,[29,30] but these changes are not often observed in melanoma. Some benign proliferations arising in congenital nevi may also manifest chromosomal aberrations by CGH, but these changes are generally different than those of melanoma.[28]

Array-based CGH has the advantage of examining the entire genome for alterations in copy number, but it requires a homogenous area of tumor cells, and there is a higher cost and longer turnaround time for results (often 3–4 weeks), at least in comparison with other technologies.[31] Recently, Ali and colleagues[32] used CGH to evaluate 10 spitzoid melanocytic lesions and reported that 9 of 10 cases had long-term clinical outcomes that correlated with the test result, whereas in 1 of 10 cases the result was uncertain. In general, sensitivity of about 92% to 96% and specificity of about 87% to 100% has been reported for the use of CGH in the diagnosis of melanoma.

## Fluorescent In Situ Hybridization

FISH is a technique that allows direct visualization of cytogenic abnormalities in cancer, such as chromosomal deletions, amplifications, and translocations.[33] Loss of heterozygosity is demonstrated by examining DNA copy number using specific loci,[34–36] and centromere-specific probes can identify gains and losses of entire chromosomes in melanomas.[37–39] FISH probes are applied directly to formalin-fixed, paraffin-embedded tissue sections, allowing assessment of interphase cells. Early cytogenic studies in melanoma identified reproducible chromosomal

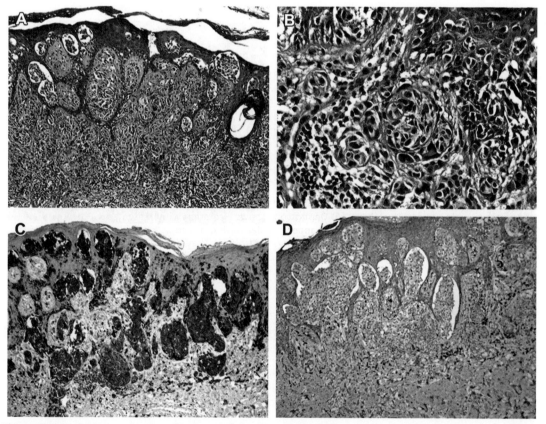

**Fig. 2.** On histologic examination, this new and changing lesion from the arm of a 25-year-old man manifested (A) irregular nesting of atypical melanocytes with pleomorphism, hyperchromasia, irregular nuclear contour, and pagetoid scatter (H&E, original magnification ×200); (B) no dermal maturation and dermal mitotic activity (circle of mitosis; original magnification ×400); (C) an equivocal proliferative index by KiMart IHC staining (MART-1 [red], Ki67 [brown], original magnification ×200); and (D) complete loss of P16 expression among melanocytes (original magnification ×200). FISH testing manifested no abnormalities, but CGH testing highlighted abnormal loss of genetic material on chromosomes 9p, 10, 19p, and 20p.

aberrations, including losses on chromosomes 6, 8, 9, and 10, and gains on chromosome 1.[27,40–43]

Although not assessing the entirety of the genome is a limitation, FISH has some advantages over CGH in some situations. FISH probes can be used on less homogenous populations of cells, and the technique is generally more expedient and of lesser cost. FISH-based detection of chromosomal abnormalities is governed by the sensitivity and specificity of the probes and technique used. Multiple probes are required for sufficient sensitivity in the diagnostic evaluation of melanocytic lesions. Often several probes, each with a distinct fluorophore, are combined into a single multicolor FISH analysis. Also, the mathematical algorithms that control detection thresholds are adjusted to impact sensitivity and specificity.

Initially, a set of four probes targeting 6p25 (RREB1), 6q23 (MYB), 11q13 (CCND1), and centromere 6 (CEP6) was offered for commercial use.[44] Positive results for melanoma were defined by the presence of one or more of the following four criteria: (1) greater than 55% nuclei with more 6p25 than CEP6 signals, (2) greater than 29% nuclei with greater than two 6p25 signals, (3) greater than 40% nuclei with fewer 6q23 than CEP6 signals, or (4) greater than 38% nuclei with greater than two 11q13 signals. These four probes have undergone evaluation in studies, with sensitivities and specificities ranging from 72% to 100% and 94% to 100%, respectively.[45–53]

However, not all parties found this original probe set (that examined only portions of chromosomes 6 and 11) to be of diagnostic utility in difficult and ambiguous melanocytic lesions.[50,54] In fact, a recent re-examination of the original probe set found three major problems in the technique: (1) low sensitivity and specificity in morphologically ambiguous melanocytic neoplasms, (2) relatively low sensitivity and specificity in spitzoid neoplasms, and (3) occurrence of false-positives caused by tetraploidy in Spitz nevi and nevus with

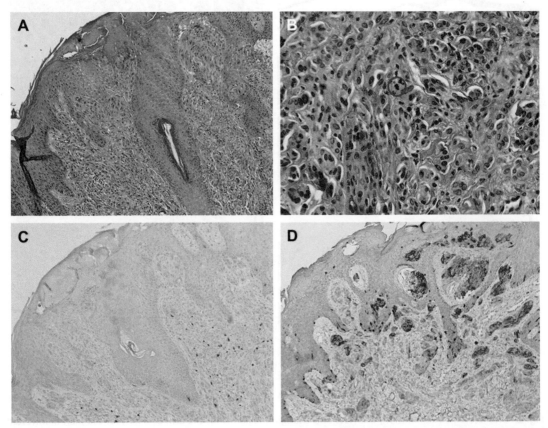

**Fig. 3.** On histologic examination, this lesion from the waistline of a 20-year-old woman manifested (*A*) atypical spitzoid cells without maturation (H&E, original magnification ×100); (*B*) deep dermal mitotic activity (*circle* of mitosis; original magnification ×400); (*C*) loss of P16 expression among all melanocytism (original magnification ×100); and (*D*) poor zonation with HMB-45 (original magnification ×100). Subsequent testing with 23-GEP manifested an abnormal (malignant) genetic signature, and limited FISH testing highlighted biallelic loss of 9p.21 (CDKN2a).

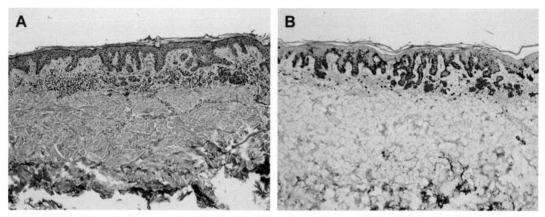

Fig. 4. GEP-2 testing using a tape stripping of a lesion from the right upper back of a 38-year-old woman demonstrated abnormal expression of LINC00518, but subsequent surgical biopsy with histologic analysis revealed only an atypical nevus, without evidence of melanoma. (*A*) H&E (original magnification ×40). (*B*) MART-1 IHC (original magnification ×40). This impression of an atypical nevus without feature of melanoma was confirmed by multiple examiners.

atypical epitheloid cell component (so-called "clonal nevi").[55] For this reason, subsequent work sought to alter the original probe set, and now the probes used typically include 9p21 (CDKN2a), 6p25 (RREB1), 11q13 (CCND1), and 8q24 (MYC).

Because of improved functionality with the addition of 11q13 and 8q24 probes, the commercial probe set from the largest single national provider (NeoGenomics, Inc, Hatfield, PA) was altered to a five-probe set consisting of 9p21 (CDKN2a), 6p25 (RREB1), 11q13 (CCND1), 8q24 (MYC), and Cen 9 (centromere of chromosome 9). Applying internally validated cutoffs, the NeoSITE Melanoma test (NeoGenomics, Inc) is reported to provide 86% sensitivity and 90% specificity, but also cases with borderline positive results can transpire, and should be interpreted with caution.

Despite the improvements made in probe constituents, exclusion of tetraploidy, and algorithm

advancement, there remain critics of the use of FISH in ambiguous lesions, particularly in those neoplasms with spitzoid features. Massi and colleagues[56] recently questioned the information gleaned from FISH testing of spitzoid neoplasm in those less than 18 years (where spitzoid lesions are more common), and no significant correlation between FISH status and clinical outcome was observed. A recent review has denounced FISH testing as a magic bullet for melanocytic processes, and instead, it has proffered that FISH represents an effective compromise "between cost, technical complexity, and diagnostic accuracy."[55]

### Case study 2

A 25-year-old man presented with a pigmented lesion of 8 × 8 mm on the left arm that had undergone growth in the last 3 months. IHC staining revealed loss of p16 among many of the cells,

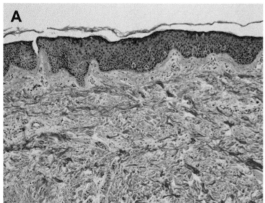
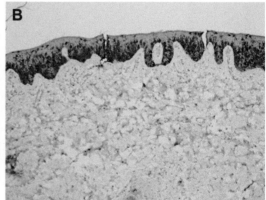

Fig. 5. GEP-2 testing using a tape stripping of a lesion from the right distal thigh of a 42-year-old woman demonstrated abnormal expression of PRAME, and subsequent surgical biopsy with histologic analysis revealed subtle melanoma in situ. (*A*) H&E (original magnification ×100). (*B*) MART-1 IHC (original magnification ×100).

**Table 1**
Comparison of melanoma assessment techniques

| Technology | Purpose | Clinical Validation | Interpretation | Clinical Impact | Practical Considerations |
|---|---|---|---|---|---|
| Histopathology | Allows for microscopic evaluation of PML to aid in diagnosis | No generalized systemic validation<br>Favorable outcome accurately predicted in 47.1% of cases, unfavorable outcome accurately predicted in 73% of cases[62] | Subjective | Histopathologic assessment of melanoma is required for AJCC staging<br>It is extremely unlikely that most institutions and insurers would proceed with care for melanoma in the absence of a histopathologic diagnosis, rendered and signed, by a licensed physician | • Gold standard for melanoma diagnosis<br>• Significant discordance among examiners |
| IHC | Adjuvant to histopathology to diagnose MM in equivocal PMLs | Sensitivity: 69%–100%<br>Specificity: unknown[16,23,63] | Objective/subjective | In PMLs with ambiguous or challenging histologic features IHC techniques may provide additional data to guide a final histologic interpretation | • Rapidity of investigations (IHC stains take only hours to perform)<br>• Cost is modest in comparison with FISH/CGH/Dx23-GEP |
| CGH | Adjuvant to histopathology to diagnose MM in equivocal PMLs | Sensitivity: 92%–96%<br>Specificity: 87%–100%[53] | Subjective | In lesions with ambiguous histologic features CGH may provide additional data to guide management | • Requires a specimen with a homogenous area of tumor cells of interest<br>• Can only provide information on increased/decreased copy numbers of genes<br>• Longer turnaround time, and generally higher costs |
| FISH | Adjuvant to histopathology to diagnose MM in equivocal PMLs | Sensitivity: 43%–100%<br>Specificity: 29%–80%[44,50,54] | Subjective | In lesions with ambiguous histologic features FISH may provide additional data to guide management | • Can only provide information on increased/decreased copy numbers of genetic material for the probe-set used<br>• Increased or decreased copy numbers outside of the probe-set yields a false-negative result<br>• Tetraploidy yields a false-positive result |

| Test | Use | Performance | Type | Comments | Notes |
|---|---|---|---|---|---|
| 23-GEP | Adjuvant to histopathology to diagnose MM in equivocal PMLs | Sensitivity: 89%–90%<br>Specificity: 91%–93%[64,65] | Objective[a] | In lesions with ambiguous histologic features DX23-GEP may provide additional data to guide management | • Validated on a small set of PMLs that included only about 10% spitzoid neoplasms<br>• Only used to differentiate between benign nevi and primary MM and subset of lesions cannot be differentiated |
| 2-GEP | Preinvasive biopsy tool used to evaluate lesions for potential surgical intervention | Sensitivity: 91%<br>Specificity: 53%–69%[66] | Objective | Because of the use of the test, as a screening device to ascertain the need for a traditional biopsy, the test has been designed to have high sensitivity, with the consequence of lesser specificity | • High sensitivity is designed to ensure that melanoma is infrequently missed by the test<br>• Lesser specificity means that some lesions that generate an abnormal result are not melanoma on surgical biopsy and histologic evaluation |
| 31-GEP | Assesses risk of metastasis in patients already diagnosed with MM | Class 1: 79%–97% 5-y DFS<br>Class 2: 31%–34% 5-y DFS[67,68] | Objective | Provides prognostic information for stage I and II melanomas, and may identify SLNBx-negative patients at additional risk for metastasis<br>May identify persons at risk for metastatic disease independent of AJCC stage, Breslow depth, ulceration status, mitotic rate, and SLNBx status[67,68] | • Requires tissue from the primary lesion<br>• Validated on a small subset of PMLs<br>• Represents an additional step in management and an additional cost to the patient |

*Abbreviation:* DFS, disease-free survival; MM, malignant melanoma; PML, problematic melanocytic lesion; SLNB, sentinel lymph node biopsy.

[a] The 23-GEP test still relies on microdissection of an area of interest from the paraffin-embedded block, and this step is subjective.

*Adapted from* the unpublished work, 2015 of the MEDTIG study group, of which the author (WA High) was a member and worked specifically on this chart.

but equivocal results with regard to assessment of the proliferative index via KiMart, and equivocal results with regard to zonation with HMB-45 (**Fig. 2**).

FISH testing with the older four-probe set (6p25 [RREB1], 6q23 [MYB], 11q13 [CCND1], and CEP6) was performed and was reported negative, whereas array-based CGH testing revealed losses of 9p, 10, 19p, and 20p. These are genetic anomalies that would not be detected with any probes in widespread commercial use (except for 9p) and it highlights the differences between FISH and CGH. The patient was judged to have melanoma and has developed regional lymph node metastases.

## TESTING MODALITIES ON THE HORIZON

One area of recent interest in melanoma diagnosis involves the activity of telomerase, an enzyme responsible for maintaining telomeric DNA during replication. Telomerase activity, in turn, is regulated by the telomerase reverse transcriptase (TERT) gene, and next-generation sequencing studies have identified mutations in the promoter of TERT (TERT-p) that increase the transcription of the gene.[57,58] TERT-p mutations have been found in 22% to 71% of cutaneous melanoma in adults, and in most conventional pediatric melanoma.[59]

Recently, investigators examined 56 patients with challenging spitzoid lesions and follow-up data for TERT-p mutations, and found four patients died of disseminated disease.[60] TERT-p mutations were detected in the four patients who developed hematogenous metastasis, but were not detected in those with favorable outcomes. TERT-p mutations were the most significant predictor of hematogenous dissemination ($P < .0001$), and it was concluded that TERT-p mutations identified a high-risk subset of patients with spitzoid neoplasms. However, other investigators reported later that although TERT-P mutations were not present in overtly benign neoplasms, such as Spitz nevi and spindle-cell nevi (of Reed), the presence of TERT-p mutations was not necessarily an adverse indicator in their series of atypical Spitz tumors and/or melanoma.[61] At present, there is no widely available genetic testing for TERT-P mutations, but additional developments in this area are anticipated.

## SUMMARY

The present state of melanoma assessment still requires histomorphologic assessment using H&E staining and light microscopy. This subjective analysis is augmented via additional data, such as IHC stain profiles or genetic testing (CGH, FISH, 23-GEP) (**Figs. 3–5**). **Table 1** summarizes the technologies used to diagnose melanoma, and some of the advantages and disadvantages of each method. Additionally, there are also new preanalytical means for identifying lesions at increased risk for being melanoma (2-GEP), which are designed to improve the biopsy selection process. Lastly, there is a new prognostic test for those patients in whom melanoma has already been assessed, and growth in this area may be reasonably anticipated as adjuvant treatment technologies and advanced surveillance protocols are developed. It is likely that the next decade will hold dramatic improvements in the ability to objectively assess and treat melanocytic lesions.

## REFERENCES

1. Musumeci G. Past, present and future: overview on histology and histopathology. J Histol Histopathol 2014;1:5.
2. Press WH. Strong profiling is not mathematically optimal for discovering rare malfeasors. Proc Natl Acad Sci U S A 2009;106:1716–9.
3. Shoo BA, Sagebiel RW, Kashani-Sabet M. Discordance in the histopathologic diagnosis of melanoma at a melanoma referral center. J Am Acad Dermatol 2010;62:751–6.
4. Hawryluk EB, Sober AJ, Piris A, et al. Histologically challenging melanocytic tumors referred to a tertiary care pigmented lesion clinic. J Am Acad Dermatol 2012;67:727–35.
5. Farmer ER, Gonin R, Hanna MP. Discordance in the histopathologic diagnosis of melanoma and melanocytic nevi between expert pathologists. Hum Pathol 1996;27:528–31.
6. McGinnis KS, Lessin SR, Elder DE, et al. Pathology review of cases presenting to a multidisciplinary pigmented lesion clinic. Arch Dermatol 2002;138:617–21.
7. Niebling MG, Haydu LE, Karim RZ, et al. Pathology review significantly affects diagnosis and treatment of melanoma patients: an analysis of 5011 patients treated at a melanoma treatment center. Ann Surg Oncol 2014;21:2245–51.
8. Patrawala S, Maley A, Greskovich C, et al. Discordance of histopathologic parameters in cutaneous melanoma: clinical implications. J Am Acad Dermatol 2016;74:75–80.
9. Bitterman A. Molecular testing to differentiate melanoma from benign nevi: the gold standard limitation. J Am Acad Dermatol 2016;75:849–50.
10. De Matos LL, Trufelli DC, de Matos MGL, et al. Immunohistochemistry as an important tool in biomarkers detection and clinical practice. Biomark Insights 2010;5:9–20.

11. Cochran AJ, Wen DR. S-100 protein as a marker for melanocytic and other tumours. Pathology 1985;17: 340–5.

12. Bishop PW, Menasce LP, Yates AJ, et al. An immuno-phenotypic survey of malignant melanomas. Histopathology 1993;23:159–66.

13. Fernando SS, Johnson S, Bate J. Immunohistochemical analysis of cutaneous malignant melanoma: comparison of S-100 protein, HMB-45 monoclonal antibody and NKI/C3 monoclonal antibody. Pathology 1994;26:16–9.

14. Kaufmann O, Koch S, Burghardt J, et al. Tyrosinase, melan-A, and KBA62 as markers for the immunohistochemical identification of metastatic amelanotic melanomas on paraffin sections. Mod Pathol 1998; 11:740–6.

15. Busam KJ. The use and application of special techniques in assessing melanocytic tumours. Pathology 2004;36:462–9.

16. Ohsie SJ, Sarantopoulos GP, Cochran AJ, et al. Immunohistochemical characteristics of melanoma. J Cutan Pathol 2008;35:433–44.

17. Jungbluth AA, Busam KJ, Gerald WL, et al. A103: an anti-melan-a monoclonal antibody for the detection of malignant melanoma in paraffin-embedded tissues. Am J Surg Pathol 1998;22:595–602.

18. Maize JC Jr, Resneck JS Jr, Shapiro PE, et al. Ducking stray "magic bullets": a Melan-A alert. Am J Dermatopathol 2003;25:162–5.

19. Nicholson KM, Gerami P. An immunohistochemical analysis of pseudomelanocytic nests mimicking melanoma in situ: report of 2 cases. Am J Dermatopathol 2010;32:633–7.

20. Vollmer RT. Use of Bayes rule and MIB-1 proliferation index to discriminate Spitz nevus from malignant melanoma. Am J Clin Pathol 2004;122: 499–505.

21. Barnhill RL. The Spitzoid lesion: rethinking Spitz tumors, atypical variants, 'spitzoid melanoma' and risk assessment. Mod Pathol 2006;19(Suppl 2): S21–33.

22. Gown AM, Vogel AM, Hoak D, et al. Monoclonal antibodies specific for melanocytic tumors distinguish subpopulations of melanocytes. Am J Pathol 1986; 123:195–203.

23. George E, Polissar NL, Wick M. Immunohistochemical evaluation of p16INK4A, E-cadherin, and cyclin D1 expression in melanoma and Spitz tumors. Am J Clin Pathol 2010;133:370–9.

24. Hilliard NJ, Krahl D, Sellheyer K. p16 expression differentiates between desmoplastic Spitz nevus and desmoplastic melanoma. J Cutan Pathol 2009;36: 753–9.

25. Harms PW, Hocker TL, Zhao L, et al. Loss of p16 expression and copy number changes of CDKN2A in a spectrum of spitzoid melanocytic lesions. Hum Pathol 2016;58:152–60.

26. Kallioniemi A, Kallioniemi OP, Sudar D, et al. Comparative genomic hybridization for molecular cytogenetic analysis of solid tumors. Science 1992; 258:818–21.

27. Bastian BC, LeBoit PE, Hamm H, et al. Chromosomal gains and losses in primary cutaneous melanomas detected by comparative genomic hybridization. Cancer Res 1998;58:2170–5.

28. Vanison C, Tanna N, Murthy AS. Comparative genomic hybridization for the diagnosis of melanoma. Eur J Plast Surg 2010;33:45–8.

29. Bastian BC, Wesselmann U, Pinkel D, et al. Molecular cytogenetic analysis of Spitz nevi shows clear differences to melanoma. J Invest Dermatol 1999;113: 1065–9.

30. Bastian BC, LeBoit PE, Pinkel D. Mutations and copy number increase of HRAS in Spitz nevi with distinctive histopathological features. Am J Pathol 2000; 157:967–72.

31. North JP, Vemula SS, Bastian BC. Chromosomal copy number analysis in melanoma diagnostics. Methods Mol Biol 2014;1102:199–226.

32. Ali L, Helm T, Cheney R, et al. Correlating array comparative genomic hybridization findings with histology and outcome in spitzoid melanocytic neoplasms. Int J Clin Exp Pathol 2010;3:593–9.

33. McCalmont TH. Gone FISHing. J Cutan Pathol 2009; 37:193–5.

34. Millikin D, Meese E, Vogelstein B, et al. Loss of heterozygosity for loci on the long arm of chromosome 6 in human malignant melanoma. Cancer Res 1991; 51:5449–53.

35. Isshiki K, Elder DE, Guerry D, et al. Chromosome 10 allelic loss in malignant melanoma. Genes Chromosomes Cancer 1993;8:178–84.

36. Isshiki K, Seng BA, Elder DE, et al. Chromosome 9 deletion in sporadic and familial melanomas in vivo. Oncogene 1994;9:1649–53.

37. Matsuta M, Kon S, Thompson C, et al. Interphase cytogenetics of melanocytic neoplasms: numerical aberrations of chromosomes can be detected in interphase nuclei using centromeric DNA probes. J Cutan Pathol 1994;21:1–6.

38. Wolfe KQ, Southern SA, Herrington CS. Interphase cytogenetic demonstration of chromosome 9 loss in thick melanomas. J Cutan Pathol 1997;24:398–402.

39. D'Alessandro I, Zitzelsberger H, Hutzler P, et al. Numerical aberrations of chromosome 7 detected in 15 microns paraffin-embedded tissue sections of primary cutaneous melanomas by fluorescence in situ hybridization and confocal laser scanning microscopy. J Cutan Pathol 1997;24:70–5.

40. Crotty KA, Scolyer RA, Li L, et al. Spitz naevus versus spitzoid melanoma: when and how can they be distinguished? Pathology 2002;34:6–12.

41. Kakati S, Song SY, Sandberg AA. Chromosomes and causation of human cancer and leukemia.

XXII. Karyotypic changes in malignant melanoma. Cancer 1977;40(3):1173–81.

42. Balaban G, Herlyn M, Guerry DT, et al. Cytogenetics of human malignant melanoma and premalignant lesions. Cancer Genet Cytogenet 1984;11:429–39.

43. Thompson FH, Emerson J, Olson S, et al. Cytogenetics of 158 patients with regional or disseminated melanoma. Subset analysis of near-diploid and simple karyotypes. Cancer Genet Cytogenet 1995;83: 93–104.

44. Gerami P, Jewell SS, Morrison LE, et al. Fluorescence in situ hybridization (FISH) as an ancillary diagnostic tool in the diagnosis of melanoma. Am J Surg Pathol 2009;33:1146–56.

45. Morey AL, Murali R, McCarthy SW, et al. Diagnosis of cutaneous melanocytic tumours by four-colour fluorescence in situ hybridisation. Pathology 2009; 41:383–7.

46. Newman MD, Lertsburapa T, Mirzabeigi M, et al. Fluorescence in situ hybridization as a tool for microstaging in malignant melanoma. Mod Pathol 2009; 22:989–95.

47. Clemente C, Bettio D, Venci A, et al. A fluorescence situ hybridization (FISH) procedure assist differentiating benign from malignant melanocytic lesions. Pathologica 2009;101:169–74.

48. Moore MW, Gasparini R. Fluorescence in-situ hybridization analysis for melanoma diagnosis. Diagn Pathol 2011;6:76–81.

49. Gerami P, Mafee M, Lurtsbarapa T, et al. Sensitivity of fluorescence in situ hybridization for melanoma diagnosis using RREB1, MYB, Cep6, and 11q13 probes in melanoma subtypes. Arch Dermatol 2010;146:273–8.

50. Vergier B, Prochazkova-Carlotti M, de la Fouchardière A, et al. Fluorescence in situ hybridization, a diagnostic aid in ambiguous melanocytic tumors: European study of 113 cases. Mod Pathol 2011;24:613–23.

51. Fang Y, Dusza S, Jhanwar S, et al. Fluorescence in situ hybridization (FISH) analysis of melanocytic nevi and melanomas: sensitivity, specificity, and lack of association with sentinel node status. Int J Surg Pathol 2012;20:434–40.

52. Abásolo A, Vargas MT, Ríos-Martín JJ, et al. Application of fluorescence in situ hybridization as a diagnostic tool in melanocytic lesions, using paraffin wax-embedded tissues and imprint-cytology specimens. Clin Exp Dermatol 2012;37:838–43.

53. Wang L, Rao M, Fang Y, et al. A genome-wide high-resolution array CGH analysis of cutaneous melanoma and comparison of array-CGH to FISH in diagnostic evaluation. J Mol Diagn 2013;15: 581–91.

54. Gaiser T, Kutzner H, Palmedo G, et al. Classifying ambiguous melanocytic lesions with FISH and

correlation with clinical long-term follow up. Mod Pathol 2010;23:413–9.

55. Ferrara G, De Vanna AC. Fluorescence in situ hybridization for melanoma diagnosis: a review and a reappraisal. Am J Dermatopathol 2016;38:253–69.

56. Massi D, Tomasini C, Senetta R, et al. Atypical Spitz tumors in patients younger than 18 years. J Am Acad Dermatol 2015;72:37–46.

57. Horn S, Figl A, Rachakonda PS, et al. TERT promoter mutations in familial and sporadic melanoma. Science 2013;339:959–61.

58. Huang FW, Hodis E, Xu MJ, et al. Highly recurrent TERT promoter mutations in human melanoma. Science 2013;339:957–9.

59. Lu C, Zhang J, Nagahawatte P, et al. The genomic landscape of childhood and adolescent melanoma. J Invest Dermatol 2015;135:816–23.

60. Lee S, Barnhill RL, Dummer R, et al. TERT promoter mutations are predictive of aggressive clinical behavior in patients with spitzoid melanocytic neoplasms. Sci Rep 2015;5:11200.

61. Requena C, Heidenreich B, Kumar R, et al. TERT promoter mutations are not always associated with poor prognosis in atypical spitzoid tumors. Pigment Cell Melanoma Res 2017;30(2):265–8.

62. Cerroni L, Barnhill R, Elder D, et al. Melanocytic tumors of uncertain malignant potential: results of a tutorial held at the XXIX Symposium of the International Society of Dermatopathology in Graz, October 2008. Am J Surg Pathol 2010;34:314–26.

63. Mason A, Wititsuwannakul J, Klump VR, et al. Expression of p16 alone does not differentiate between Spitz nevi and Spitzoid melanoma. J Cutan Pathol 2012;39:1062–74.

64. Clark LE, Warf MB, Flake DD, et al. Clinical validation of a gene expression signature that differentiates benign nevi from malignant melanoma. J Cutan Pathol 2015;42(4):244–52.

65. Clarke LE, Berking C, Tahan S, et al. Development of a gene expression signature to differentiate malignant melanoma from benign melanocytic nevi. Poster presentation: Society for Melanoma Research International Congress. Philadelphia, November 17–19, 2013.

66. Gerami P, Yao Z, Polsky D, et al. Development and validation of a noninvasive 2-gene molecular assay for cutaneous melanoma. J Am Acad Dermatol 2017;76(1):114–20.e2.

67. Gerami P, Cook RW, Wilkinson J, et al. Development of a prognostic genetic signature to predict the metastatic risk associated with melanoma. Clin Cancer Res 2015;21(1):175–81.

68. Gerami P, Cook RW, Russell MC, et al. Gene expression profiling for molecular staging of cutaneous melanoma in patients with sentinel lymph node biopsy. J Am Acad Dermatol 2015;72(5):780–5.e3.

# Assessing Genetic Expression Profiles in Melanoma Diagnosis

Sancy A. Leachman, MD, PhD[a],*,
Stephanie Mengden Koon, MD[b],
Veselina B. Korcheva, MD[b], Kevin P. White, MD[b]

## KEYWORDS

- GEP • RT-PCR • Genetic expression profiling • Diagnostic test • Melanoma

## KEY POINTS

- Genetic expression profiling (GEP) is an emerging diagnostic tool used to assist in discrimination between benign nevi and malignant melanomas.
- GEP evaluates a panel of genes with reverse transcription quantitative polymerase chain reaction to determine if mRNA expression is more consistent with a benign or malignant pattern.
- GEP tests face challenges with respect to demonstration of improvement upon the current pathologic "gold standard" for diagnosis of melanoma.
- National Comprehensive Cancer Network Guidelines do not recommend use of GEP diagnostic assays for routine clinical care.
- Like fluorescent in situ hybridization and array comparative genomic hybridization technologies, GEP may supply additional, independent information regarding challenging or ambiguous lesions; results should be considered in the context of the histopathologic findings, on a case-by-case basis.

## INTRODUCTION

Accurate diagnosis of melanoma is critical. Thin melanomas have a better prognosis than thick melanomas,[1] presumably because they represent earlier lesions that do not have the biological capacity to metastasize. Thus, if appropriately treated, most thin melanomas are curable. In contrast, most advanced melanomas are lethal, despite recent advances in targeted immunotherapies. Most melanocytic tumors can be readily categorized as benign or malignant with traditional histopathology. However, there is a subset of ambiguous/equivocal melanocytic tumors with the potential to metastasize that defy classification with conventional histologic criteria. The interobserver reproducibility among pathologists in the evaluation of challenging melanocytic neoplasms is also poor.[2–5] Thus, the "gold-standard" histologic evaluation has the potential to miss a subset of lethal melanomas.

The consequences of missing these ambiguous, yet lethal melanomas are dire and frequently result

Disclosure Statement: Dr S.A. Leachman received honoraria and travel expenses of less than $5000 over the last 5 years from Myriad Genetic Laboratories for participating as a Medical and Scientific Advisory Board member. She has also participated in Myriad's early access programs for Myriad myPath and myRisk genetic tests. Drs S. Mengden Koon, V.B. Korcheva, and K.P. White have no conflicts of interest with respect to this article.
[a] Melanoma and Skin Cancer Program, Department of Dermatology, OHSU Knight Cancer Institute, Oregon Health & Science University, 3303 SW Bond Avenue, Portland, OR 97239, USA; [b] Department of Dermatology, Oregon Health & Science University, 3303 SW Bond Avenue, Portland, OR 97239, USA
* Corresponding author. Center for Health and Healing, 3303 Southwest Bond Avenue, Suite 16 D, Portland, OR 97239.
E-mail address: leachmas@ohsu.edu

Dermatol Clin 35 (2017) 537–544
http://dx.doi.org/10.1016/j.det.2017.06.016
0733-8635/17/© 2017 The Authors. Published by Elsevier Inc. This is an open access article under the CC BY-NC-
ND license (

in more aggressive, morbid, costly procedures and treatments, and death in some cases. In addition, the medicolegal risk has reinforced the need for providers to err on the side of caution.[6,7] For these reasons, there has been a drift in the diagnostic criteria that may increase sensitivity of melanoma detection, at the expense of specificity.[8–12] This shift toward cautious behavior may protect the patient and providers from misdiagnosis, but may also lead to overtreatment and a disproportionate increase in melanoma incidence rates relative to mortalities.[13] Ideally, a diagnostic test that exceeds the current gold standard would be more objective and increase reproducibility and specificity without compromising sensitivity.

## MOLECULAR DIAGNOSTIC TESTS FOR MELANOMA

One candidate diagnostic tool is genetic expression profiling (GEP; **Table 1**). GEP is a relatively recent addition to the diagnostic armamentarium for melanoma and differs from DNA-based testing such as fluorescent in situ hybridization (FISH) and comparative genomic hybridization (CGH) (tumor cytogenetics). Over the past decade, ambiguous melanocytic tumors have been increasingly evaluated using FISH and/or CGH (see **Table 1**). FISH has the advantage of evaluating for large chromosomal deletions, duplications, and translocations in a subset of chromosomal loci that have a well-established association with melanoma.[14] However, only a limited number of chromosomal loci are evaluated; the interpretation remains subjective, and specialized expertise is required.[15] CGH overcomes some, but not all, of the subjectivity of FISH and allows evaluation of large chromosomal aberrations across the entire genome.[16,17] However, CGH requires relatively large quantities of tissue and is limited by tumor heterogeneity, making it less reliable in thinner neoplasms.[17] Although FISH and CGH are the most commonly used molecular diagnostic tests to date, GEP is an alternative molecular technology that could improve diagnostic accuracy, by increasing objectivity, reducing variability, and taking advantage of changes in the tumor's biology. **Table 1** summarizes the most salient features of the various diagnostic tests for melanocytic lesions.

## GENETIC EXPRESSION PROFILING METHODOLOGY
### Tissue Collection

GEP is a relatively straightforward method used to detect abnormal expression of messenger RNA (mRNA). Ideally, the assay will follow Minimum

Information for Publication of Quantitative Real-Time PCR Experiments (MIQE) Guidelines.[36] GEP uses reverse transcription in combination with quantitative polymerase chain reaction (RT-qPCR) technology (**Fig. 1**). The whole tumor (including the surrounding stromal microenvironment) or a dissected or a laser-captured component can be tested, using fresh, frozen, or formalin-fixed and paraffin-embedded tissue. Microdissection allows an enriched collection of malignant cells and improves the sensitivity by reducing contamination with benign cells. Conversely, use of the undissected tumor has the advantage of capturing expression changes induced in the tumor microenvironment, for example, normal stromal and inflammatory cells.

### Reverse Transcription of Messenger RNA to complementary DNA

Once tumor tissue is obtained, RNA is extracted and complementary DNA (cDNA) is created from mRNA using RT. Multiple factors can affect this step, including the source of RT, variability in the quantity and quality of the tumor RNA, mRNA priming methods, and even reaction protocols. Therefore, using standardized reagents and protocols and mandating quality assurance of the tissues and tested RNA is paramount. Otherwise, process variability may exceed the differences observed in gene expression between benign and malignant lesions, leading to an invalid test. Testing the quality and quantity of cDNA is also important because accurate quantification of gene expression requires RT and qPCR reactions to occur in a linear range.

### Quantitative Expression Analysis

After sufficient cDNA is obtained, genes selected for the expression profile are amplified by using gene-specific primers, designed to amplify the genes of interest with qPCR (MIQE Guidelines suggest the primer sequence, or at least the region of the gene being amplified, to be made available in publications). The amplification process is measured in real time, and through comparison to a set of coamplified control genes, determines how much mRNA from each gene was present in the original sample. Internal control genes and standardized RNA extraction kits, primer construction, and PCR equipment have reduced variability in this step. Reliable analytical methods exist for quantifying expression; however, detailed information regarding the testing protocol remains critical. In some cases, protocol details are considered proprietary, making independent validation of the test challenging.

**Table 1**
Comparison of diagnostic tests for melanoma

| Test | Analytical Validation (Reproducibility) | Clinical Validation | | Interpretation | Clinical Utility (Utilization of Results) | Performance vs Outcomes |
|---|---|---|---|---|---|---|
| | | Performance | Reference Standard | | | |
| Histopathology | 38% discordance rate among experts reviewing "classic" examples of melanocytic neoplasms[5] | No general systematic validation against outcomes performed; discordance rate for melanocytic tumors varies from 15% to 50% Favorable outcome accurately predicted in 47.1% of cases, unfavorable outcome accurately predicted in 73% of cases[18] | Clinical follow-up $\geq$5 y[18] | Subjective | No systematic study of pathology report recommendations vs actual treatment performed | *Favorable outcome:* Accurately predicted in 47.1% of cases *Unfavorable outcome:* Accurately predicted in 73% of cases[18] |
| IHC | Variability of IHC has been widely documented[19–25] | Sensitivity: 69%–100%, Spec: uncertain[26] | Histopathology[26] | Subjective | Changed diagnosis in 11% of all lesions; confirmed or excluded differential diagnosis in 77%[27] | N/A |
| FISH | Clinical validation not published, but required to be on file for CLIA-certified laboratories | Sensitivity range: 43%–100%, specificity range: 29%–80%[14,28,29] | Pathologists within the same institutions that developed the test[14] | Subjective | 88% of cases received a more definitive diagnosis[30] | Sensitivity: 100% Specificity: 71% for 21 Outcome-proven cases[14] |
| aCGH | Clinical validation not published, but required to be on file for CLIA-certified laboratories | Sensitivity range: 92%–96%, specificity range: 87%–100%[16,17] | Institution's original pathology report[16,17] | Subjective | Not published to date | 9/10 cases had outcomes that matched aCGH result, 1/10 results was uncertain[31] |
| GEP | 2.5% SD[32] | Sensitivity: 90%,[33] 91.5%,[34] Specificity: 91%,[33] 92.5%[34] | Concordant diagnoses by 2–3 independent pathologists[33,34] | Objective | 49.1% change in treatment recommendations[35] | TBD |

*Abbreviations:* aCGH, array comparative genomic hybridization; IHC, immunohistochemistry; N/A, not available; TBD, to be determined.

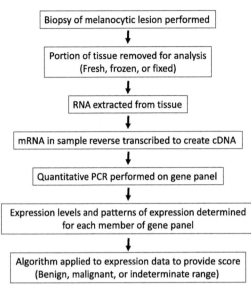

**Fig. 1.** GEP methodology for melanoma diagnosis. The methodology for GEP is relatively straightforward as shown. Critical elements for a successful clinical assay include rigorous standardization and quality assurance of each technical step, careful selection of the gene panel, and independent validation of the assay.

### Scoring Algorithms

Mathematical models and algorithms can be developed to create an objective scoring system. This modeling allows gene expression data to be normalized and weighted according to the importance of the genes with respect to malignant behavior. Weighting is based on known function or on data about a specific gene's influence on the benign or malignant state. Alternatively, gene selection can be agnostic, based on data obtained during the discovery phase of the assay. The scoring metric produces a numeric result for each sample that classifies it into a benign, malignant, or indeterminate range and eliminates the need for expert interpretation. However, the specific model must be tested in independent sample sets in order to be validated and may require evolution in order to maximize accuracy over time.

### Gene Selection

Selection of GEP genes is crucial for the success of the assay. The genes in the melanoma GEP panel are differentially expressed in benign versus malignant tumors. The rationale is that malignant behavior of a tumor is permitted (and/or driven) by increases or decreases in expression of certain genes compared with their expression in a benign state. This approach may be more powerful than

FISH or CGH in identifying malignant lesions because it measures a functional consequence of malignant transformation rather than the mutation or mutations that drives the change. If key mRNA indicators of transformation can be identified and measured, these genes can be used to create a melanoma expression signature (a process known as discovery). That signature must then be verified in a large and diverse set of human tissue samples, confirming that the differences in expression levels of the genes are statistically significant. It must then be clinically validated using an independent (nonoverlapping) set of samples (a cohort that does not include any samples used previously). Ideally, the results of the initial clinical validation will then be confirmed using additional, larger, multi-institutional, prospectively obtained sets of samples collected through a uniform, reproducible protocol. The gene panel validation studies should demonstrate sensitivity and specificity that improves upon current diagnostic methods and supports inclusion as a clinical test.

## CHALLENGES IN GENETIC EXPRESSION PROFILING DESIGN AND VALIDATION
### Specimen Variability

Limitations exist with respect to GEP validation. Adequately annotated tumor samples may not be available for development and validation of the assay. Tissue archives may not be available for research purposes. Older samples may not provide acceptable quality of RNA. Sufficient material for GEP testing may be limited in small melanocytic tumors. Taken together, these issues may result in the need to combine specimens from several archives to test or validate the assay. Utilizing multiple specimens can potentially increase the variability in the results given the lack of uniform handling of the samples.

In addition, interpathologist variability may lead to diagnostic differences such that a lesion read as a severely atypical nevus by some might be classified by others as melanoma in situ. Furthermore, melanoma may represent a small portion of the tissue, and little or no melanoma may be left for GEP testing. For these reasons, centralized pathology review is appropriate before GEP testing.

### Candidate Genes Are Often Identified in a Nonambiguous Sample Set

In order to select genes that are differentially expressed, with the potential to discriminate between benign and malignant melanocytic tumors, the original discovery is often performed on samples that are unequivocally benign and malignant.

Ambiguous/equivocal lesions are assumed to lie along a biological continuum that is intermediate between benign nevi and melanoma and will share molecular changes with both ends of the spectrum (have intermediate mRNA expression patterns) for which a cutoff can ultimately be assigned. However, it is possible that some ambiguous/equivocal lesions differ at the molecular level from their nonambiguous counterparts.

If the biology of the ambiguous/equivocal lesion is different from the neoplasms used in discovery and verification, it is possible that the lesion may also have a different GEP. Therefore, a critical step in validating a diagnostic GEP for evaluation of ambiguous or equivocal melanocytic lesions is validation in a large, adequately powered set of these ambiguous/equivocal lesions, including those with special features and behaviors.

### Ambiguous/Equivocal Specimen Analysis Is Complex

There are several challenges associated with validating a GEP assay in an ambiguous/equivocal sample set. All previously noted caveats (see earlier discussion under Specimen variability) apply. It may be difficult to obtain enough "ambiguous" cases. Furthermore, one pathologist's "ambiguous lesion" may represent another's obvious melanoma. One approach to define diagnostic ambiguity is to document the interobserver variability among pathologists; however, this standard is seldom applied to large cohorts for practical reasons.

The ultimate goal of a melanoma GEP assay is to accurately identify melanocytic lesions with metastatic potential so that they can be adequately treated *and* to identify nonlethal lesions that do not necessitate further treatment. Without a definitive diagnosis, equivocal lesions are nearly always treated *as if* they are malignant. Removal of these lesions interrupts the natural history of the tumor, and so a failure to metastasize is not informative (ie, the lesion might have been benign, or it could have been malignant but was treated before metastasis by its removal). It is therefore difficult if not impossible to "prove" that a lesion is benign. Rare cases do exist in which ambiguous/equivocal melanocytic lesions (1) are not reexcised and recur with a malignant phenotype, or (2) are not reexcised and metastasize, or (3) are reexcised but still recur and/or metastasize. These rare cases are extremely informative, but difficult to identify or to obtain for research purposes.

### Establishing a New Gold Standard

In addition to the above challenges, a major obstacle exists with respect to improving upon the histology-based "gold standard." This difficulty is in part because a pathologic diagnosis was used to develop the assay. Genes are selected as markers of "benign" or "malignant" based on their capacity to recapitulate the pathologists' assignments of benign or malignant. Therefore, it is not surprising that GEP shows high specificity and sensitivity in unambiguous lesions as measured by the histologic gold standard. However, if sensitivity or specificity decreases when the GEP is applied to ambiguous/equivocal lesions, it is difficult to know if the assay failed to provide the correct result or if the pathologist failed to provide the correct diagnosis. The only way to ascertain whether the pathologic assessment has been improved upon by a GEP assay is to follow these cases over time and determine if the GEP predicted malignant recurrences or metastases that were not anticipated based on histology. As discussed above, this progression is rare, and validation by this method will be difficult.

### Myriad myPath Genetic Expression Profiling for Melanoma

Promising GEP markers for the diagnosis of melanoma were identified and published in 2005, and have been identified in laser-microdissected melanomas.[37,38] Currently, only one GEP diagnostic test for melanoma is available on the market, a 23-gene expression signature developed by Myriad Genetic Laboratories. The assay measures gene expression and generates a score that falls within a range considered benign, malignant, or indeterminate. The signature is marketed under the name Myriad myPath Melanoma and it has undergone 2 independent clinical validation studies across a variety of histologic subtypes.[33,34] The National Comprehensive Cancer Network Guidelines for Melanoma Version 2.2016, a states: "While there is interest in newer prognostic molecular techniques such as gene expression profiling to differentiate benign from malignant neoplasms, or melanomas at risk for low versus high-risk of metastasis, routine (baseline) genetic testing of primary cutaneous melanomas (before or following sentinel lymph node biopsy) is not recommended outside of a clinical study (trial)." This footnote within the melanoma guidelines seems to be primarily directed toward prognostic GEP testing, but this nonprofit alliance of 27 leading national cancer centers advises caution with respect to considering any GEP test as a new standard of care. A recent publication by Cockerell and colleagues[35] demonstrated, however, that dermatopathologists were significantly influenced by the GEP with respect to the diagnosis and recommendations rendered. As with FISH and CGH, there may be a role for the GEP assay in providing additional information regarding lesions that are not easily interpreted with traditional histopathology.

## SUMMARY

When is it acceptable to transition a new diagnostic test into the clinical realm? On one hand, it would be ideal to know as much as possible about the true sensitivity and specificity of the new assay with respect to long-term outcomes such as recurrence, metastasis, and death. However, is it appropriate to deprive patients of the technology while waiting for this type of confirmatory evidence that will take years to obtain? As with many aspects of medicine, the application of new tools and technologies requires both a scientific rigor and a more intuitive appreciation of where the tool may be helpful. Although a GEP melanoma diagnostic cannot yet be considered standard of care for every melanocytic lesion, there are ambiguous cases in which a provider may feel the extra information provided by the test is helpful.

## REFERENCES

1. Balch CM, Gershenwald JE, Soong SJ, et al. Final version of 2009 AJCC melanoma staging and classification. J Clin Oncol 2009;27(36):6199–206. Available at: https://www.ncbi.nlm.nih.gov/pmc/articles/PMC2793035/pdf/zlj6199.pdf.

2. Nobre AB, Pineiro-Maceira J, Luiz RR. Analysis of interobserver reproducibility in grading histological patterns of dysplastic nevi. An Bras Dermatol 2013;88(1):23–31. Available at: https://www.ncbi.nlm.nih.gov/pmc/articles/PMC3699937/pdf/abd-88-0023.pdf.

3. Hawryluk EB, Sober AJ, Piris A, et al. Histologically challenging melanocytic tumors referred to a tertiary care pigmented lesion clinic. J Am Acad Dermatol 2012;67(4):727–35. Available at: http://ac.els-cdn.com/S0190962212002678/1-s2.0-S0190962212002678-main.pdf?_tid=38eeddb2-d2bf-11e6-b0dc-00000aab0f6c&acdnat=1483563121_df3311cbce05c50a780e97da45af1117.

4. Braun RP, Gutkowicz-Krusin D, Rabinovitz H, et al. Agreement of dermatopathologists in the evaluation of clinically difficult melanocytic lesions: how golden is the 'gold standard'? Dermatology 2012;224(1):51–8. Available at: https://www.karger.com/Article/Pdf/336886.

5. Farmer ER, Gonin R, Hanna MP. Discordance in the histopathologic diagnosis of melanoma and melanocytic nevi between expert pathologists. Hum Pathol 1996;27(6):528–31. Available at: https://www.ncbi.nlm.nih.gov/pubmed/?term=8666360.

6. Troxel DB. Pitfalls in the diagnosis of malignant melanoma: findings of a risk management panel study. Am J Surg Pathol 2003;27(9):1278–83. Available at: http://ovidsp.tx.ovid.com/ovftpdfs/FPDDNCFBIEOEKP00/fs042/ovft/live/gv020/00000478/00000478-200309000-00012.pdf.

7. Troxel DB. Trends in pathology malpractice claims. Am J Surg Pathol 2012;36(1):e1–5. Available at: http://ovidsp.tx.ovid.com/ovftpdfs/FPDDNCFBIEOEKP00/fs047/ovft/live/gv024/00000478/00000478-201201000-00001.pdf.

8. Frangos JE, Duncan LM, Piris A, et al. Increased diagnosis of thin superficial spreading melanomas: a 20-year study. J Am Acad Dermatol 2012;67(3):387–94. Available at: http://ac.els-cdn.com/S0190962211011832/1-s2.0-S0190962211011832-main.pdf?_tid=8aefa78e-d2c1-11e6-838b-00000aacb360&acdnat=1483564118_2b279dc7cc3a088fdeb0c7220daf43e3.

9. Carney PA, Frederick PD, Reisch LM, et al. How concerns and experiences with medical malpractice affect dermatopathologists' perceptions of their diagnostic practices when interpreting cutaneous melanocytic lesions. J Am Acad Dermatol 2016;74(2):317–24 [quiz: 324.e1–8]. Available at: http://ac.els-cdn.com/S0190962215022355/1-s2.0-S0190962215022355-main.pdf?_tid=865c7b70-d2c1-11e6-838b-00000aacb360&acdnat=1483564110_d512abe6cb8181715337e571168b148a.

10. Marsch A, High WA. Medicolegal issues with regard to melanoma and pigmented lesions in dermatopathology. Dermatol Clin 2012;30(4):593–615, v–vi. Available at: http://ac.els-cdn.com/S0733863512000812/1-s2.0-S0733863512000812-main.pdf?_tid=918c9dea-d2c1-11e6-acf9-00000aab0f02&acdnat=1483564129_13b5fd76a05ddf37688906efba94cca5.

11. Brenn T. Pitfalls in the evaluation of melanocytic lesions. Histopathology 2012;60(5):690–705. Available at: http://onlinelibrary.wiley.com/store/10.1111/j.1365-2559.2011.04042.x/asset/j.1365-2559.2011.04042.x.pdf?v=1&t=ixjfnqxd&s=33051857a8b9ac89b2b5d7600a46c3c82474a75d.

12. Moshell AN, Parikh PD, Oetgen WJ. Characteristics of medical professional liability claims against dermatologists: data from 2704 closed claims in a voluntary registry. J Am Acad Dermatol 2012;66(1):78–85. Available at: http://ac.els-cdn.com/S0190962210021560/1-s2.0-S0190962210021560-main.pdf?_tid=8ea25bec-d2c1-11e6-98f0-00000aab0f26&acdnat=1483564124_ca7f1244e536795d65e34746d8e3f30d.

13. SEER Stat Fact Sheets: Melanoma of the Skin. Division of Cancer Control and Population Sciences Surveillance Research Program. Available at: https://seer.cancer.gov/statfacts/html/melan.html.

14. Gerami P, Jewell SS, Morrison LE, et al. Fluorescence in situ hybridization (FISH) as an ancillary diagnostic tool in the diagnosis of melanoma. Am J Surg Pathol 2009;33(8):1146–56. Available at: http://ovidsp.tx.ovid.com/ovftpdfs/FPDDNCLBFANJHB00/fs047/ovft/live/gv031/00000478/00000478-2009080 00-00004.pdf.

15. Busam KJ. Molecular pathology of melanocytic tumors. Semin Diagn Pathol 2013;30(4):362–74. Available at: http://www.sciencedirect.com/science/article/pii/S0740257013000464.

16. Bastian BC, Olshen AB, LeBoit PE, et al. Classifying melanocytic tumors based on DNA copy number changes. Am J Pathol 2003;163(5):1765–70. Available at: https://www.ncbi.nlm.nih.gov/pmc/articles/PMC1892437/pdf/3846.pdf.

17. Wang L, Rao M, Fang Y, et al. A genome-wide high-resolution array-CGH analysis of cutaneous melanoma and comparison of array-CGH to FISH in diagnostic evaluation. J Mol Diagn 2013;15(5):581–91. Available at: http://ac.els-cdn.com/S15251 57813000925/1-s2.0-S1525157813000925-main.pdf?_tid=fce0c72e-d2c1-11e6-8ec6-00000aacb35e&acdnat=1483564309_e23ec16465ef97761f404baa 78266162.

18. Cerroni L, Barnhill R, Elder D, et al. Melanocytic tumors of uncertain malignant potential: results of a tutorial held at the XXIX Symposium of the International Society of Dermatopathology in Graz, October 2008. Am J Surg Pathol 2010;34(3):314–26. Available at: http://ovidsp.tx.ovid.com/sp-3.23.1b/ovidweb.cgi?WebLinkFrameset=1&S=BFICFPJCEEDDB JMNNCHKGHJCECBJAA00&returnUrl=ovidweb.cgi%3f%26Full%2bText%3dL%257cS.sh.18.19% 257c0%257c00000478-201003000-00003%26S% 3dBFICFPJCEEDDBJMNNCHKGHJCECBJAA00& directlink=http%3a%2f%2fovidsp.tx.ovid.com% 2fovftpdfs%2fFPDDNCJCGHMNEE00%2ffs047% 2fovft%2flive%2fgv031%2f00000478%2f00000478- 201003000-00003.pdf&filename=Melanocytic+ Tumors+of+Uncertain+Malignant+Potential%3a+ Results+of+a+Tutorial+Held+at+the+XXIX+ Symposium+of+the+International+Society+of+ Dermatopathology+in+Graz%2c+October+2008. &pdf_key=FPDDNCJCGHMNEE00&pdf_index=/ fs047/ovft/live/gv031/00000478/00000478-2010030 00-00003.

19. El Shabrawi-Caelen L, Kerl H, Cerroni L. Melan-A: not a helpful marker in distinction between melanoma in situ on sun-damaged skin and pigmented actinic keratosis. Am J Dermatopathol 2004;26(5):364–6. Available at: http://ovidsp.tx.ovid.com/sp-3.23.1b/ovidweb.cgi?WebLinkFrameset=1&S=ONIM FPICGNDDBJKDNCHKLFLBIBGEAA00&returnUrl= ovidweb.cgi%3f%26Full%2bText%3dL%257cS.sh. 18.19%257c0%257c00000372-200410000-00003% 26S%3dONIMFPICGNDDBJKDNCHKLFLBIBGE AA00&directlink=http%3a%2f%2fovidsp.tx.ovid. com%2fovftpdfs%2fFPDDNCLBLFKDGN00% 2ffs047%2fovft%2flive%2fgv031%2f00000372% 2f00000372-200410000-00003.pdf&filename= Melan-A%3a+Not+a+Helpful+Marker+in+ Distinction+between+Melanoma+In+Situ+on+ Sun-Damaged+Skin+and+Pigmented+Actinic+ Keratosis.&pdf_key=FPDDNCLBLFKDGN00&pdf_ index=/fs047/ovft/live/gv031/00000372/00000372- 200410000-00003.

20. Maize JC Jr, Resneck JS Jr, Shapiro PE, et al. Ducking stray "magic bullets": a Melan-A alert. Am J Dermatopathol 2003;25(2):162–5. Available at: http://ovidsp.tx.ovid.com/ovftpdfs/FPDDNCFBIEOE KP00/fs024/ovft/live/gv013/00000372/00000372- 200304000-00013.pdf.

21. Beltraminelli H, Shabrawi-Caelen LE, Kerl H, et al. Melan-a-positive "pseudomelanocytic nests": a pitfall in the histopathologic and immunohistochemical diagnosis of pigmented lesions on sun-damaged skin. Am J Dermatopathol 2009;31(3):305–8. Available at: http://ovidsp.tx.ovid.com/ ovftpdfs/FPDDNCFBIEOEKP00/fs047/ovft/live/gv031 /00000372/00000372-200905000-00018.pdf.

22. Argenyi ZB, Cain C, Bromley C, et al. S-100 protein-negative malignant melanoma: fact or fiction? A light-microscopic and immunohistochemical study. Am J Dermatopathol 1994;16(3):233–40.

23. Busam KJ, Chen YT, Old LJ, et al. Expression of melan-A (MART1) in benign melanocytic nevi and primary cutaneous malignant melanoma. Am J Surg Pathol 1998;22(8):976–82.

24. Fullen DR, Reed JA, Finnerty B, et al. S100A6 preferentially labels type C nevus cells and nevic corpuscles: additional support for Schwannian differentiation of intradermal nevi. J Cutan Pathol 2001;28(8):393–9. Available at: https://deepblue.lib. umich.edu/bitstream/handle/2027.42/75660/j.1600- 0560.2001.028008393.x.pdf?sequence=1.

25. King R, Google PB, Weilbaecher KN, et al. Microphthalmia transcription factor expression in cutaneous benign, malignant melanocytic, and nonmelanocytic tumors. Am J Surg Pathol 2001; 25(1):51–7. Available at: http://ovidsp.tx.ovid.com/ sp-3.23.1b/ovidweb.cgi?WebLinkFrameset=1&S= FHJFFPICPMDDBJFENCHKLDFBPMPDAA00& returnUrl=ovidweb.cgi%3f%26Full%2bText%3dL% 257cS.sh.18.19%257c0%257c00000478-20010 1000-00005%26S%3dFHJFFPICPMDDBJFENCH KLDFBPMPDAA00&directlink=http%3a%2f%2 fovidsp.tx.ovid.com%2fovftpdfs%2fFPDDNCFBLD FEPM00%2%ffs028%2fovft%2flive%2fgv009%2f00 000478%2f00000478-200101000-00005.pdf&file name=Microphthalmia+Transcription+Factor+ Expression+in+Cutaneous+Benign%2c+Malignant +Melanocytic%2c+and+Nonmelanocytic+Tumors. &pdf_key=FPDDNCFBLDFEPM00&pdf_index=

/fs028/ovft/live/gv009/00000478/00000478-20010
1000-00005.

26. Ohsie SJ, Sarantopoulos GP, Cochran AJ, et al. Immunohistochemical characteristics of melanoma. J Cutan Pathol 2008;35(5):433–44. Available at: http://onlinelibrary.wiley.com/store/10.1111/j.1600-0560.2007.00891.x/asset/j.1600-0560.2007.00891.x.pdf?v=1&t=ixl02hi0&s=89c26e35dc9061cc7f1b fca6782837978e3b5868.

27. Naert KA, Trotter MJ. Utilization and utility of immunohistochemistry in dermatopathology. Am J Dermatopathol 2013;35(1):74–7. Available at: http://ovidsp.tx.ovid.com/ovftpdfs/FPDDNCFBIEOEKP00/fs047/ovft/live/gv024/00000372/00000372-201302 000-00011.pdf.

28. Gaiser T, Kutzner H, Palmedo G, et al. Classifying ambiguous melanocytic lesions with FISH and correlation with clinical long-term follow up. Mod Pathol 2010;23(3):413–9. Available at: http://www.nature.com/modpathol/journal/v23/n3/pdf/modpathol2009 177a.pdf.

29. Vergier B, Prochazkova-Carlotti M, de la Fouchardiere A, et al. Fluorescence in situ hybridization, a diagnostic aid in ambiguous melanocytic tumors: European study of 113 cases. Mod Pathol 2011;24(5):613–23. Available at: http://www.nature.com/modpathol/journal/v24/n5/full/modpathol2010 228a.html.

30. North JP, Garrido MC, Kolaitis NA, et al. Fluorescence in situ hybridization as an ancillary tool in the diagnosis of ambiguous melanocytic neoplasms: a review of 804 cases. Am J Surg Pathol 2014;38(6): 824–31. Available at: http://ovidsp.tx.ovid.com/sp-3.23.1b/ovidweb.cgi?WebLinkFrameset=1&S= MJHEFPHCBPDDBJJBNCHKFFLBFFGPAA00& returnUrl=ovidweb.cgi%3f%26Full%2bText%3dL% 257cS.sh.18.19%257c0%257c00000478-2014060 00-00011%26S%3dMJHEFPHCBPDDBJJBNCHKFF LBFFGPAA00&directlink=http%3a%2f%2fovidsp.tx. ovid.com%2fovftpdfs%2fFPDDNCLBFFJBBP00% 2ffs047%2fovft%2flive%2fgv024%2f00000478% 2f00000478-201406000-00011.pdf&filename= Fluorescence+In+Situ+Hybridization+as+an+ Ancillary+Tool+in+the+Diagnosis+of+Ambiguous +Melanocytic+Neoplasms%3a+A+Review+of+ 804+Cases.&pdf_key=FPDDNCLBFFJBBP00&pdf _index=/fs047/ovft/live/gv024/00000478/00000478-201406000-00011.

31. Ali L, Helm T, Cheney R, et al. Correlating array comparative genomic hybridization findings with histology and outcome in spitzoid melanocytic neoplasms. Int J Clin Exp Pathol 2010;3(6):593–9. Available at: https://www.ncbi.nlm.nih.gov/pmc/articles/PMC2907121/pdf/ijcep0003-0593.pdf.

32. Warf MB, Flake DD 2nd, Adams D, et al. Analytical validation of a melanoma diagnostic gene signature using formalin-fixed paraffin-embedded melanocytic lesions. Biomark Med 2015;9(5):407–16. Available at: http://onlinelibrary.wiley.com/doi/10.1111/cup.12475/abstract;jsessionid=961C277829E54F4 A96153D005650D48A.f03t02.

33. Clarke LE, Warf MB, Flake DD 2nd, et al. Clinical validation of a gene expression signature that differentiates benign nevi from malignant melanoma. J Cutan Pathol 2015;42(4):244–52. Available at: http://onlinelibrary.wiley.com/store/10.1111/cup.12475 /asset/cup12475.pdf?v=1&t=ixjfux1a&s=6ba1d2 936b62fc7e8dbff44a32a5f52d89dd5a83.

34. Clarke LE, Flake DD 2nd, Busam K, et al. An independent validation of a gene expression signature to differentiate malignant melanoma from benign melanocytic nevi. Cancer 2016;123(4):617–28. Available at: http://onlinelibrary.wiley.com/store/10.1002/cncr.30385/asset/cncr30385.pdf?v=1&t=ixjfuqvl&s =6732c6a273e97e7b0a7b6a16f0e13ad036a0f714.

35. Cockerell CJ, Tschen J, Evans B, et al. The influence of a gene expression signature on the diagnosis and recommended treatment of melanocytic tumors by dermatopathologists. Medicine 2016;95(40):e4887. Available at: https://www.ncbi.nlm.nih.gov/pmc/articles/PMC5059047/pdf/medi-95-e4887.pdf.

36. Bustin SA, Benes V, Garson JA, et al. The MIQE guidelines: minimum information for publication of quantitative real-time PCR experiments. Clin Chem 2009;55(4):611–22. Available at: http://clinchem. aaccjnls.org/content/clinchem/55/4/611.full.pdf.

37. Torabian S, Kashani-Sabet M. Biomarkers for melanoma. Curr Opin Oncol 2005;17(2):167–71. Available at: http://ovidsp.tx.ovid.com/ovftpdfs/FPDDNCLBFANJHB00/fs047/ovft/live/gv031/00001 622/00001622-200503000-00016.pdf.

38. Jaeger J, Koczan D, Thiesen HJ, et al. Gene expression signatures for tumor progression, tumor subtype, and tumor thickness in laser-microdissected melanoma tissues. Clin Cancer Res 2007;13(3):806–15. Available at: http://clincancerres.aacrjournals.org/content/clincanres/13/3/806.full.pdf.

# Assessing Genetic Expression Profiles in Melanoma Prognosis

Aaron S. Farberg, MD[a],*, Alex M. Glazer, MD[b],
Richard R. Winkelmann, DO[c], Darrell S. Rigel, MD, MS[d]

## KEYWORDS

- Skin cancer • Melanoma • Prognosis • DecisionDx-melanoma • Genetic expression profile

## KEY POINTS

- A 31-genetic expression profile (31-GEP) test to predict metastatic risk of melanoma has been previously validated and classifies patients as either class 1 (low risk) or class 2 (high risk).
- The 31-GEP in combination with other prognostic characteristics or tools (American Joint Committee on Cancer online tool and sentinel lymph node biopsy) provides superior prognostic capability.
- Clinical utilization studies reveal the 31-GEP test had a significant and appropriate impact on management while remaining within the context of established guidelines.
- Limited follow-up data required to correlate the 31-GEP with outcomes are available. The 31-GEP has not been included in any official guideline recommendations, either as standard of care or as part of clinical trials.

## INTRODUCTION

The incidence of cutaneous malignant melanoma (CMM) has continued to increase, and although it accounts for less than 5% of all skin cancers, it causes the greatest number of skin cancer–related deaths worldwide.[1] Following a diagnosis of CMM, patients are classified by the American Joint Committee on Cancer (AJCC) system that defines CMM staging.[2] A patient's staging status in conjunction with national guidelines can then be used for subsequent evidenced-based management by their dermatologist.

Despite advances in management and treatment, the factor that most impacts prognosis remains early detection of the malignancy that is responsible for the detection of thinner CMM lesions at diagnosis. Although it is well demonstrated that Breslow thickness predicts disease-free survival and overall survival, other potential characteristics have been evaluated for the prognosis of patients with CMM.[3]

Currently, the following clinical and pathologic prognostic markers of CMM are incorporated for clinical use: Breslow thickness, presence of ulceration, presence of microsatellites, and regional lymph node involvement.[2] Mitotic rate is included only for melanomas ≤1 mm in thickness. Unfortunately, even after decades of research on various prognostic markers, the guideline recommendations are often similar across several tumor stages in part because of their inability to stratify different

Disclosure Statement: Dr A.S. Farberg: Served as a consultant to Castle Biosciences Inc. Dr A.M. Glazer: Participated in a research fellowship that was partially funded by Castle Biosciences Inc. Dr R.R. Winkelmann: None. Dr D.S. Rigel: Served as a consultant to Castle Biosciences Inc.

[a] Department of Dermatology, Icahn School of Medicine at Mount Sinai, 5 East 98th Street, Floor 5, New York, NY 10029, USA; [b] National Society for Cutaneous Medicine, New York, NY 10016, USA; [c] Ohio Health, Columbus, OH 43214, USA; [d] New York University Medical Center, New York, NY 10016, USA

* Corresponding author.

E-mail address: aaron.farberg@gmail.com

derm.theclinics.com

risk groups that may have markedly different outcomes.[4,5]

The difficulties in discretely stratifying CMM staging are apparent. Although sentinel lymph node biopsy (SLNB) has been shown to be the most accurate independent prognostic parameter in CMM, positive SLNB status only identifies one-third of patients with CMM who develop metastatic disease and ultimately die.[6,7] The SLNB negative patients are generally managed with lower intensity strategies that include less frequent physician-patient interaction, yet 2 out of 3 patients who die from melanoma are initially diagnosed with stage I and II disease, and most recurrences (up to 70%) are detected by the patient.[6,8] Furthermore, prognosis for clinical stage II and III cases by TNM is highly variable, as evidenced by a 5-year survival rate of 53% to 82% for stage II patients and a 5-year survival rate of 22% to 68% for stage III patients.[2,7] Although the use of prognostic factors in conjunction with staging is a strong predictor of metastatic spread, the clinical use of each factor has limitations.

Several new molecular tests for melanoma have been developed that are based on gene expression patterns from RNA obtained from formalin-fixed paraffin-embedded sections from the biopsy specimens of lesions. These molecular techniques provide information that cannot be gleaned from clinical or histologic examination and may provide significant prognostic capability.

A 31-genetic expression profile (31-GEP) test (DecisionDx-Melanoma, Castle Biosciences Inc, Friendswood, TX, USA) was developed as a diagnostic test to assist physicians in the management of CMM.[9] Based on a patient's primary tumor expression levels of a panel of genes, a lesion is classified as either "low risk" (class 1) or "high risk" (class 2) for metastasis. The 31-GEP has significant potential to affect clinical practice in the management of CMM.

## CONTENT
### 31-Genetic Expression Profile Test

The quantitative reverse transcription polymerase chain reaction–based 31-GEP test is obtained from samples that are collected from formalin-fixed paraffin-embedded CMM tissue and arranged in 5-μm sections on microscope slides.[9] RNA isolation is performed followed by an assessment of its quality and quantity. The RNA is then converted to complementary DNA and undergoes amplification before being loaded to microfluidics gene cards containing primers specific for the 31 gene targets. The gene expression assay is performed in triplicate. Radial basis machine predictive modeling is performed, which is a nonlinear classification based on the normalized values for each gene. The modeling transforms the gene measurements using a kernel function to find an optimal hyperplane in multivariate dimension, thus providing a predicted classification of high and low risk tumor biology.

### Initial Development and Validation

For the development of the 31-GEP, Gerami and colleagues[9] used published genomic analysis of CMM tumors to determine a unique prognostic genetic signature for metastatic risk. Genes were selected on the basis of significant genetic expression variation in metastatic and nonmetastatic CMM across several published studies. Of 54 identified genes, the investigators selected 20 based on chromosomal location. Genes from a similar uveal melanoma panel were added in addition to specific BAP1 gene probes. A signature comprising 28 prognostic genetic targets and 3 control genes was developed from the expression data. The 31-GEP was applied to 268 primary CMM cases (collected from 7 independent centers) with clinical follow-up of at least 5 years unless there was a well-documented metastatic event, including positive SLNB.

The study initially reported the use of the test to predict metastasis in patients diagnosed with stage I or II CMM using an independent validation set consisting of 104 cases.[9] Of these cases, 35 had developed metastatic disease, and there was median follow-up of 7.3 years for the cases that did not. The 5-year disease-free survival was 97% among the 61 cases with a class 1 "low-risk" signature and 31% for the 43 cases with a class 2 "high-risk" signature. Negative predictive value and positive predictive value were 93% and 72%, respectively. The receiver operating characteristic curve was 0.91 for the validation set and 0.93 for the original training set, which is consistent with a clinically relevant predictive model.

For stage I and II cases in the validation set that had either a metastatic event or more than 5 years of follow-up without metastasis, class 1 disease-free survival was 98% compared with class 2 with a rate of 37%.[9] Median follow-up for cases in this cohort was 7.6 years. When combined, the validation and training cohorts consisted of 220 stage I and II CMM cases. Overall, the 31-GEP accurately identified 120 of 134 (90%) stage I/IIA cases without documented evidence of metastasis as class 1 (low risk) and 24 of 30 (80%) stage I/IIA cases with documented metastasis as class 2 (high risk) (sensitivity, 90%; specificity, 84%; positive predictive value = 72%; negative predictive value = 95%).

When compared with other AJCC staging criteria, regression analysis characterized the 31-GEP as a strong independent predictor of metastatic risk along with Breslow thickness, ulceration, age, and higher level of staging.[9] The initial 31-GEP development and validation study revealed the test to be an independent and powerful prognosticator of metastasis in stage I and II CMM patients.

### 31-Genetic Expression Profile and American Joint Committee on Cancer Online Prognostic Tool

The AJCC Individualized Melanoma Outcome Prediction Tool Web-based prognostic tool is often used by clinicians to attain survival rate estimates and appropriate management recommendations.[10] In a separate follow-up study, Ferris and colleagues[11] compared the accuracy of the 31-GEP test with the accuracy of the AJCC Web-based prognostic tool. For the evaluation, two 5-year overall survival rate cutoffs (79% and 68%) were used because they reflect the 5-year survival rates for CMM stage IIA (79%) and stage IIB (68%). These stages were chosen because patients in these cohorts can receive significantly different surveillance and treatment based upon national guidelines.[4,5] These rates were used as cutoff scores to establish low- and high-risk groups based on the AJCC-predicted outcomes, which were then compared with the 31-GEP results.

Two hundred five stage I and II CMMs were used in the comparison.[11] Univariate analysis revealed significant risk assessment for all 3 predictors (31-GEP, AJCC 79%, and AJCC 68%). Determination of risk was significantly correlated with recurrence, distant metastasis, and death. Multivariate regression indicated that the 31-GEP is more significantly associated with the endpoints of distant metastasis and death. The 31-GEP also had a significantly higher sensitivity, but lower specificity when compared with the AJCC predictor at both cutoff scores.

The 31-GEP classification combined with the AJCC prognostic tool enhanced sensitivity, reflecting a more accurate identification of high-risk stage I and II melanoma patients.[11] The combination predictor resulted in accurate identification of 90% of cases with recurrences, 88% of distant metastases, and 82% of deaths. Multivariate analysis comparing the combined 31-GEP and AJCC tools also outperformed risk prediction by the AJCC tool alone.

### 31-Genetic Expression Profile and Sentinel Lymph Node Biopsy

The predictive accuracy of the 31-GEP and SLNB was evaluated individually and in combination in order to assess disease-free survival, distant metastasis-free survival, and overall survival. Two hundred seventeen invasive CCM samples from patients who also underwent the SLNB procedure were analyzed using the 31-GEP test in a multicenter prospective study.[12] Of the 58 patients with a positive SLNB, 37 (64%) experienced a metastatic event, 32 (55%) developed distant metastasis, and 18 (31%) died of all causes. The 31-GEP test identified 141 cases as class 2 (high risk), of which 91 (65%) progressed to metastatic disease. Seventy-one (50%) developed distant metastasis, and 53 (38%) died of all causes. Although both SLNB and the 31-GEP were found to be significant predictors on Cox regression, for each end point the 31-GEP had a higher hazard ratio compared with SLNB ($P<.0001$).

Combining the 31-GEP test and SLNB status further improved metastatic risk prognostication.[12] This combination is particularly valuable because the 2 tests may identify patients at high risk for recurrence who otherwise would have been classified as lower risk. The study showed this for the 42% of patients who had a 31-GEP class 2 (high risk) but a negative SLNB. For this group, the 5-year disease-free, metastasis-free, and overall survival were 35%, 49%, and 54%, respectively. These rates were not different from the subset of patients who were class 2 with a positive SLNB. When used in combination with SLNB, the 31-GEP may help clinicians identify high-risk SLNB-negative patients with aggressive disease.

A major limitation of this study was that the overall risk of metastatic events was about 30% higher in the SLNB-negative cohort of patients than is usually found in the general CMM population.

### Clinical Utility

Although the 31-GEP has demonstrated reproducibility and clinical validity in assessing recurrence risk, another important aspect is clinical utility: the impact of the test results on clinical decision making. Three unique prospective studies have evaluated the management changes of clinicians using the 31-GEP test.

One study reviewed 156 CMM patients who were consecutively 31-GEP tested from 6 institutions (3 dermatology and 3 surgical oncology practices) to evaluate the clinical impact and influences on physicians directing management.[13] Frequency of clinical visits, frequency and modality of imaging, SLNB procedure utilization, referrals, and frequency of blood laboratory work was compared. Changes in management were observed in 82 (53%) patients with most class 2 patients (77%) undergoing management changes compared with only 37% of class 1 patients (*P*<.0001). The majority (77/82, 94%) of these changes were concordant with the risk indicated by the 31-GEP test result with increased management intensity for class 2 patients and reduced intensity for class 1 patients. Similar significant risk-appropriate changes were found in frequency of office visits and use of advanced imaging (PET/computed tomography).

An important finding of this utilization study was the minimal effect of the 31-GEP on recommendation and use of SLNB.[13] Only 2 of the 156 cases had a change in SLNB utilization for which the procedure was performed. However, both cases were 31-GEP class 1, which suggests other factors prompted the modified management. For patients that underwent SLNB (112), the 31-GEP test results appeared impactful on subsequent management. Ninety-nine patients (89%) had a negative result. Within this group, 55 patients were class 1; 27 (49%) patients had a reduction in the intensity of their management, whereas none had an increase. Forty-four of the patients were class 2; 35 (80%) of these patients were given increased management intensity. Although the utility of the 31-GEP test in combination with SLNB status had shown value in prognostication,[12] the test now has shown physicians are able to individualize patient management by increasing or decreasing surveillance according to each patient's clinical presentation.

Two separate studies also evaluated the 31-GEP clinical utility by dermatologists using patient vignettes. Dermatology resident physicians (n = 169) responded to a series of questions asking to identify the Breslow thickness at which decisions about SLNB, imaging, and oncology referrals would be made.[14] Additional responses were obtained about willingness to use SLNB procedure or imaging based on patient vignettes with variable clinical characteristics. Answers for all questions were compared when class 1, class 2, or no 31-GEP test result information was provided.

When the 31-GEP test results were not provided, most respondents adhered to current management guidelines for recommending SLNB.[14] The addition of the 31-GEP test information led to significant risk-appropriate changes in management decisions. A class 2 result had an impact on SLNB, imaging, and oncology referral in 47%, 50%, and 47% of physician respondents where

as a class 1 result led to a change in only 23%, 18%, and 19%. Similar results were found for the vignettes, where a class 1 designation resulted in a significant decrease in recommendations for SLNB and imaging, but an appropriate increase for class 2 results.

Although the resident physician study showed the 31-GEP may appropriately impact clinical decision making, the test was also evaluated by board-certified dermatologists who may be more cautious in adopting newer technology. Similar results were found for the effects of the 31-GEP in clinical management in their study of 214 dermatologists (Glazer AM, et al. Submitted for publication). In their inflection point analysis, a class 2 result caused 69% and 61% of respondents to choose a thinner Breslow thickness of 0.7 mm for recommending SLNB and imaging. The Breslow thickness inflection point selected to guide SLNB and imaging was changed by a class 1 result (41% and 32%, respectively) and class 2 result (66% and 67%, respectively). Interestingly, the experienced dermatologists were more willing to modify patient management than the resident physicians when incorporating the results of the 31-GEP test.

## Limitations and Technical Issues

Molecular testing has been used for prognostic purposes, but the clinical use of these methods has been limited by their susceptibility to sampling error resulting from tumor heterogeneity, limited clinical validation, lack of standardized testing, and high technical failure rates. The development and validation set included 268 patients followed by multiple subsequent validations studies. These results have allowed dermatologists to augment management of CMM patients, but given the toxicity of adjuvant therapy, further validation may be needed before oncologists responsible for treating patients with advanced disease use the test in a significant manner. Furthermore, the test does not currently have a role in determining which patients are candidates for adjuvant immunotherapy, either as a standard of care or as part of clinical trials.

The impact of the 31-GEP results on health outcomes may also be further evaluated. Although the endpoint of the utilization study was to analyze changes in clinical management resulting from class assignments, the study was limited by the absence of follow-up data required to correlate the 31-GEP with outcomes.[13] Future studies would benefit from the collection of follow-up data to show the impact of clinical practice adjustments on patient outcomes.

Although there is great promise, the 31-GEP has not been included in any national or professional association guideline recommendations. If the 31-GEP continues to prove to be an accurate predictor of metastasis, the test may guide decision making regarding staging procedures and adjuvant therapy.

## SUMMARY

Providing an accurate estimate of prognosis is a fundamental goal in the management of all melanoma patients. Physicians can inform patients of their probable clinical course, thereby facilitating clinical management recommendations. It is also essential for optimizing the design and evaluation of clinical trials as well.

Novel therapeutic advances in melanoma treatment continue to occur to improve the outcomes for subsets of patients. Identifying those who would derive benefit as well as those who could be spared from the potentially morbid or costly therapy will be important from the perspective of both a patient and a health care system.

The 31-GEP test has significant potential to affect clinical practice in the management of CMM. The most acute utility appears in helping to identify aggressive tumors and adjust management accordingly. Having the additional molecular information to identify patients that do not appear to be at higher risk for metastasis but may, in fact, be so due to genetic factors, will be clinically useful. The enhanced sensitivity of detecting more aggressive subtypes would allow for enhanced surveillance and earlier therapeutic intervention all to the benefit of the patient.[15] However, the particular impact for the 31-GEP is still incompletely defined. Other substantial impacts include downstaging of management and prediction of tumor biologic behavior. Such applications will require additional validation by clinical trials with additional CMM samples and long-term clinical follow-up.

A summary of current published peer-reviewed studies evaluating the 31-GEP can be found in **Table 1**. Validation studies have shown the 31-GEP result to be significant clinical information that can be used in combination with the AJCC online tool or SLNB to improve stratification of patients with CMM, thereby allowing the opportunity for improved patient treatment. Utilization of the 31-GEP allowed individualized management based on biological risk while still remaining within the context of established practice guidelines for melanoma patient management. The integration of the 31-GEP as an emerging prognostic factor into previously validated melanoma prognostic tools represents an important challenge that must be met for such tools to remain clinically relevant.

**Table 1**
**Summary of current published peer-reviewed studies evaluating the 31-genetic expression profile**

| Study | Study Type | Sample Size | Conclusions |
|---|---|---|---|
| Gerami et al,[9] 2015 | Retrospective multicenter | 268 | Development and validation of the independent prognostic accuracy of 31-GEP |
| Gerami et al,[12] 2015 | Retrospective multicenter | 217 | 31-GEP was more accurate in prognosis than SLNB; however, combination of 31-GEP/SLNB status was superior |
| Ferris et al,[11] 2016 | Retrospective multicenter | 205 | 31-GEP provides prognostic information and improves identification of high-risk CMM when used in combination with AJCC online tool |
| Berger et al,[13] 2016 | Prospective cohort multicenter | 156 | 31-GEP augments clinical management consistent with risk appropriate manner |
| Farberg et al,[14] 2017 | Utilization survey | 169 | 31-GEP had significant and appropriate impact on management by resident physician dermatologists |
| Glazer AM, et al. Submitted for publication | Utilization survey | 214 | 31-GEP had significant and appropriate impact on management by board-certified dermatologists |

## REFERENCES

1. Siegel RL, Miller KD, Jemal A. Cancer statistics, 2016. CA Cancer J Clin 2016;66:7–30.
2. Balch CM, Gershenwald JE, Soong SJ, et al. Final version of 2009 AJCC melanoma staging and classification. J Clin Oncol 2009;27:6199–206.
3. Mandala M, Massi D. Tissue prognostic biomarkers in primary cutaneous melanoma. Virchows Arch 2014;464:265–81.
4. Coit DG, Thompson JA, Algazi A, et al. Melanoma, Version 2.2016, NCCN Clinical Practice Guidelines in Oncology. J Natl Compr Canc Netw 2016;14(4): 450–73.
5. Bichakjian CK, Halpern AC, Johnson TM, et al. Guidelines of care for the management of primary cutaneous melanoma. American Academy of Dermatology. J Am Acad Dermatol 2011;65(5): 1032–47.
6. Morton DL, Thompson JF, Cochran AJ, et al. Final trial report of sentinel-node biopsy versus nodal observation in melanoma. N Engl J Med 2014;370: 599–609.
7. Balch CM, Gershenwald JE, Soong SJ, et al. Multivariate analysis of prognostic factors among 2,313 patients with stage III melanoma: comparison of nodal micrometastases versus macrometastases. J Clin Oncol 2010;28:2452–9.
8. Morton DL, Thompson JF, Cochran AJ, et al. Sentinel-node biopsy or nodal observation in melanoma. N Engl J Med 2006;355:1307–17.
9. Gerami P, Cook RW, Wilkinson J, et al. Development of a prognostic genetic signature to predict the metastatic risk associated with cutaneous melanoma. Clin Cancer Res 2015;21:175–83.
10. v7 AJCC melanoma database. Available at: www. melanomaprognosis.org. Accessed December 5, 2016.
11. Ferris LK, Farberg AS, Middlebrook B, et al. Identification of high risk cutaneous melanoma tumors is improved when combining the online AJCC melanoma patient outcome prediction tool with a 31-gene expression profile–based classification. J Am Acad Dermatol 2016;76(5):818–25.e3.
12. Gerami P, Cook RW, Russell MC, et al. Gene expression profiling for molecular staging of cutaneous melanoma in patients with sentinel lymph node biopsy. J Am Acad Dermatol 2015;72:780–5.
13. Berger AC, Davidson RS, Poitras JK, et al. Clinical impact of a 31-gene expression profile test for cutaneous melanoma in 156 prospectively and consecutively tested patients. Curr Med Res Opin 2016; 32(9):1599–604.
14. Farberg AS, Glazer AM, White R, et al. Impact of a 31-gene expression profiling test for cutaneous melanoma on dermatologists' clinical management decisions. J Drugs Dermatol 2017;16(5):428–31.
15. Podlipnik S, Carrera C, Sanchez M, et al. Performance of diagnostic tests in an intensive follow-up protocol for patients with American Joint Committee on Cancer (AJCC) stage IIB, IIC, and III localized primary melanoma: a prospective cohort study. J Am Acad Dermatol 2016; 75(3):516–24.

# Smartphone-Based Applications for Skin Monitoring and Melanoma Detection

Elizabeth Chao, MD, PhD[a], Chelsea K. Meenan, BS[b],
Laura K. Ferris, MD, PhD[a],*

## KEYWORDS

- Smartphone • Mobile app • Teledermatology • Mobile teledermoscopy • Malignant melanoma
- Skin cancer screening • Regulatory oversight

## KEY POINTS

- Smartphone applications (apps) offer a unique approach to enhance the delivery of dermatologic care.
- Despite the abundance of apps in skin cancer education and screening, few have been evaluated for clinical efficacy and none has been sufficiently accurate and reliable using established research methodologies.
- The US Food and Drug Administration (FDA) has proposed guidelines to regulate mobile apps, but there are currently no established quality standards or regulatory oversight of mobile medical apps to ensure patient safety and minimize harm.
- The wide availability of smartphone apps has raised important ethical concerns regarding patient confidentiality, informed consent, transparency of data ownership, and data privacy protection.
- Further studies are needed to assess the safety and efficacy of smartphone medical apps as diagnostic tools in skin cancer screening.

## INTRODUCTION

According to a 2015 Pew Research Center report, 92% of US adults own a cell phone and 68% have a smartphone, up from 35% in 2011, with smartphone ownership nearing the saturation range of 83% to 86% for adults ages 18 to 49.[1] As smartphones have rapidly gained popularity, there are now thousands of available mobile medical apps available, with a considerable number of these apps developed in dermatology, where clinical diagnosis is largely based on visual examination. Although these apps have potential to offer novel pathways to deliver health care, there are concerns regarding their safety, confidentiality, quality of content, and regulation. Hamilton, Brady and March and colleagues[2,3] surveyed 229 dermatology-related apps, with those relevant to melanoma or skin cancer spanning a spectrum of functions, including reference or educational aids, self-surveillance and diagnostic tools, teledermatology, and research. More than half of the apps are free of charge, with paid apps ranging in price from $0.99 to

Disclosures: L.K. Ferris has developed and published data on a melanoma detection classifier although this is not commercialized. E. Chao and C.K. Meenan have no conflicts to declare.
a Department of Dermatology, University of Pittsburgh Medical Center, Pittsburgh, PA 15213, USA; b School of Medicine, University of Pittsburgh, Pittsburgh, PA 15213, USA
* Corresponding author. 3601 Fifth Avenue, 5th Floor, Pittsburgh, PA 15213.
E-mail address: ferrislk@upmc.edu

Dermatol Clin 35 (2017) 551–557
http://dx.doi.org/10.1016/j.det.2017.06.014
0733-8635/17/© 2017 Elsevier Inc. All rights reserved.

$139.99, with a median price of $2.99. Only 33% of app descriptions explicitly stated a named dermatologist and 31% claimed involvement of doctors or a medical team whereas in 36% of apps, authorship information was not disclosed.[2] Moreover, a case study evaluating the accuracy of 4 apps to correctly classify 60 melanoma and 128 benign control lesions found the results highly variable with three-fourths of the apps incorrectly classifying 30% or more of the melanoma lesions.[4]

This article presents a review and characterization of various types of smartphone-based apps for skin monitoring and melanoma detection for use by the general public. The list of apps actually available at a given time changes daily so the focus is on app categories with examples, along with some of their potential advantages and pitfalls (**Table 1**). Progress toward regulatory body–approved and scientifically evaluated mobile health apps with an update of current FDA regulation in the field of medical apps, as well as ethical challenges currently affecting the field are also discussed.

## PATIENT EDUCATION

To date, a majority of smartphone apps aimed at melanoma detection serve primarily as an educational resource for patients, providing information about melanoma and/or skin cancer, sun protection recommendations based on skin type and UV radiation exposure, and instruction on skin self-examination and use of the asymmetry, border, color, diameter, evolution (ABCDE) method for evaluation of moles.[2,5] Surprisingly, the development of only a few apps have involved the input of dermatologists,[6] and most apps lack disclosure of authorship and credentials, which are often not readily available within the primary description.[2]

Educational apps for the general population provide users information on melanoma and other skin cancers, such as *ABCDEs of Melanoma* or *Melanoma iABCD rule*. Other apps provide more general dermatologic information, such as *Dermatology A to Z*, offered by the American Academy of Dermatology that provides information about dermatologic conditions, gives the current UV index, and offers links to find a dermatologist in the area. One of the most widely reviewed mobile apps is *Ultraviolet ~ UVIndex*, which tailors sun protection recommendations based on location as determined by a global positioning system. There are also smartphone apps targeted toward specific patient populations, such as *Skin Care for Transplant Recipients*, which provides educational materials, photographic atlas and skin self-examination tutorial, mole mapping, a UV-B index, appointment reminders, and list of transplant specialists for follow-up care for solid organ transplant recipients.

Despite the abundance of educational apps, only a few have been evaluated for clinical efficacy to date. *Solar Cell*, the first sun safety mobile app evaluated in a randomized clinical trial, delivers personalized real-time sun protection education to help individuals make informed decisions regarding sun exposure and sun protection.[7,8] Unfortunately, the results of the study were largely disappointing because the app was not only unable to exhibit any impact on reducing sunburn prevalence but also was associated with decreased sunscreen use. The study exposed 2 major pitfalls of mobile-based health interventions: (1) sustained behavioral change is challenging and cannot be achieved in isolation with apps and (2) most individuals who download apps fail to use them regularly.

## SELF-SURVEILLANCE AND TOTAL BODY DIGITAL PHOTOGRAPHY

More than half of all dermatologic smartphone apps provide patients with self-monitoring capabilities, including tools to log, organize, and track their concerning moles using their mobile device's built-in camera. This allows patients to communicate with providers regarding potential concerns. Self-surveillance apps vary in their capabilities, with some allowing patients to document lesions, follow diagnostic algorithms, log personal treatment regimens, or record symptoms. *UMSkinCheck*, an app developed by the University of Michigan, as well as *LoveMySkinMole map*, *FotoSkin*, and *Embarrassing Bodies – My MoleChecker*, are apps that allow users to compile a digital image library of moles and other relevant lesions. *ApreSkin* takes documentation one step further by using a 3-D model to mark and record moles.

Mole mapping has been shown a useful tool for dermatologists to improve the accuracy of melanoma detection. Patients can also benefit from using their digital images to detect new and changing nevi during their skin self-examinations. Not surprisingly, apps designed to aid the user in collecting a set of digital mole mapping images are also available. One such example is *CompariSkin*. Given the sensitive nature of these photos, privacy and security of such images is a major concern. *DermaCompare* is one of the few melanoma detection apps whose cloud is reported to be Health

**Table 1**
**Smartphone applications for skin cancer monitoring and detection: Pros and Cons**

| Smartphone Application Type | Pros | Cons |
|---|---|---|
| Educational—provides information on skin cancer diagnosis and/or risk factors | • Inexpensive way to educate across wide geographic area<br>• Simple to update<br>• Minimal potential for risk to patient | • Audience limited to those with smartphones and knowledge of technology<br>• No process to verify quality and accuracy of information |
| Mole mapping—allows patients to take images of either individual moles of concern or to take own set of full-body digital images | • Inexpensive<br>• Patient can use at home to collect own images<br>• Easy for patient to use images during skin self-examination | • Variable image quality<br>• Not useful for physician during screenings in office<br>• Risk of security breech if stored on app's server vs patient phone |
| Teledermatology—provides platform for patient-directed teledermatology | • Some apps are inexpensive<br>• Access to dermatologist for patients with financial, time, geographic barriers<br>• May be good option for routine follow-up in established dermatologist-patient relationship<br>• Some apps integrate teledermatology visit into patients electronic medical record<br>• Can integrate patient-performed teledermoscopy for appropriate high-risk patients | • Limited health insurance coverage<br>• Not all treating physicians are dermatologists or licensed in a patient's state of residence<br>• Many apps do not adhere to standards of high-quality telemedicine<br>• Risk of poor-quality images if taken by patient with a smartphone<br>• Not all guarantee adequate protection of protected health information |
| Diagnostic—allows user to collect image of suspicious lesion and uses internal algorithm to perform a risk assessment for a lesion | • May raise awareness, encourage patients to seek medical attention<br>• Potential for future development using validated algorithms<br>• Inexpensive | • Currently no regulatory oversight<br>• No quality standards<br>• Risk of falsely reassuring patient that a skin cancer is benign and delaying diagnosis of skin cancer or causing unnecessary anxiety if wrong |
| Research—allows individuals to participate in research studies using their smartphone | • Can reduce research expenses by allowing informed consent, photos, clinical information to be entered via smartphone<br>• Access to research participants nationwide<br>• Can integrate smartphone sensors for data collection<br>• Use of available ResearchKit by Apple facilitates design and addresses data security concerns<br>• Can anonymize data and share with wider research community | • Limit to data that can be collected with a smartphone (no blood, tissue, genetic data)<br>• Cannot validate patient-reported data in most cases<br>• Limited ability to provide intervention via smartphone |

Insurance Portability and Accountability Act (HIPAA) compliant. Many dermatologic smartphone apps, however, lack capabilities for secure photo storage during total-body digital photography–guided skin examinations by patients.[9] Although self-monitoring has the potential to be an effective health behavior intervention, the effort required to track an individual's moles can present a significant barrier to sustained use. Some apps, including

*MySkinPal* and *SelfCheck*, offer push reminders to patients to perform self-checks monthly, but it is not known if this has in impact on skin self-examination rates.

## DIRECT-TO-PATIENT TELEDERMATOLOGY

Telemedicine is a rapidly evolving method of health care delivery that has also expanded to utilize mobile technologies as a platform to deliver both direct-to-patient teledermatology and, more recently, patient-directed teledermoscopy. This is likely attributable to the advancement of smartphones with high-resolution built-in digital cameras and high-speed Internet connectivity and the development of dermatoscopes that can be paired with smartphones. In addition, geographic, economic, and time barriers limit access to dermatologists for some patients and teledermatology offers a potential solution to this problem.[10]

Strictly mobile-based teledermatology services now comprise approximately 8% to 10% of direct-to-consumer teledermatology practices.[6,11] Costs per consult are priced similarly to other teledermatology services, averaging approximately $40 to $100, with one app, *DermCheck*, offering a monthly subscription of $20/month for unlimited concierge dermatology access. Although these services can be used to address a wide variety of dermatologic conditions, evaluation of lesions suspicious for skin cancer is one primary application of this technology.

Smartphone apps follow a direct patient care model by enabling patients to initiate a consultation with a dermatologist without a prior referral. They primarily use a store-and-forward methodology, a form of asynchronous consultation where a patient transmits his/her medical history and digital images for review by a dermatologist who within a prespecified timeframe provides consultative review and appropriate treatment.

Some teledermatology apps primarily focus on offering a medical opinion about skin lesions suspicious for skin cancer. One example is *Mole Doctor Skin Cancer App Dermatologist*, which costs $9.99 and gives an opinion in 24 hours. Although the name suggests the opinion is from a dermatologist, the app information only states the opinion will be from a "real doctor." Studies show variable diagnostic accuracy of teledermatology and teledermoscopy compared with face-to-face visits, but in some cases accuracy is comparable.[12] A recent study of direct-to-consumer teledermatology platforms, however, found that many did not provide the identity and credentials of the consulting physician or used physicians who were not licensed to practice medicine in the state of the patient or even in the United States. The same study found that 3 of 14 consultants failed to correctly identify a nodular melanoma as concerning and that adherence to teledermatology guideline, such as offering a choice of physicians and providing a report back to a patient's primary care physician, was rare.[13] Thus, the quality of the service provided is often dubious.

Another concern about mobile teledermatology apps is the lack of privacy measures and policies. This is particularly concerning in cases when sensitive photos may be submitted and when the treating physician or provider is outside the United States. Compounding this is the ability of most smartphones to track personal information, such as a user's location. Although some mobile apps, such as *First Derm*, avoid this issue by offering full anonymity, this violates established teledermatology guidelines. Only a few apps, such as *DermEngine*, *SkyMD*, and *Spruce*, specify a privacy clause in their mobile platform. Many of these apps do not meet the criteria for high-quality teledermatology proposed by the American Academy of Dermatology.[14]

New to the field of teledermatology is patient-directed teledermoscopy. One app, *MoleScope*, works together with a small dermatoscope that costs $99, fits on a smartphone, and can be used by a patient to capture dermatoscopic images that can then be shared with a dermatologist. Although studies have shown that this strategy is potentially feasible and acceptable to patients,[15] it is not widespread in use, requires specialized tools, and is likely best suited for high-risk patients whose dermatologists are comfortable with this modality.

## AUTOMATED LESION ASSESSMENT AND RISK CLASS

Not all dermatologic medical apps utilize physicians for assessment of skin lesions and melanoma. Some assess lesions using a mathematical algorithm and provide an assessment using a risk stratification system. The risk stratification described by such apps categorizes lesions as low risk, medium risk, or high risk by using pattern recognition software comparing a database of nevi with confirmed melanoma diagnoses to patient images. Apps use their own algorithm and grading scale to assess risk and typically provide a recommendation corresponding with the risk assessment. *DoctorMole*, is a self-surveillance app that not only saves images of lesions, allowing users to compare changes over time, but also provides a risk assessment of each mole. Additionally, apps like *skinScan*, categorize high-risk lesions, accompanied by a recommendation to see a physician soon, whereas medium-risk and low-risk lesions are recommended to be tracked and shown to physicians during annual skin checks.

Apps that provide lesion assessments and risk classification offer users guidance regarding the degree of urgency to seek medical attention for a lesion. Thus, these apps work to triage patients. Unfortunately, this can lead to missed diagnoses with false risk assessment, giving users a false sense of security about potentially lethal lesions or causing unnecessary worry if a benign lesion in misclassified.[4] The consequences of this can be grave, particularly if treatment of a melanoma is delayed because of an app's assessment.

## USE OF APPLICATIONS FOR RESEARCH IN SKIN CANCER

With the introduction of Apple's ResearchKit, smartphones that have the ability to collect photographs as well as biometric and clinical data that can be used in research. Utilizing a mobile app for research purposes allows researchers to eliminate geographic barriers, increase assessment frequency with ease of communication and access to participants, and reduce enrollment costs by coordinating participation through an online interface. One research app, Mole Mapper, allows users to tracks moles over time, allowing patients to see changes in size to share with their medical team and to participate in active melanoma research by transmitting images and answers to questions about melanoma risk factors to researchers for analysis. Uses can provide informed consent to participate in research via the app.

The use of apps for research also has inherent limitations. One limitation of app-based research is selection bias because only patients who own and are facile with the use of smartphones can participate. Another limitation is the inability of researchers to validate patient-reported findings independently. Additionally, because the mode of participation is solely by mobile apps, research studies have limits in design, such as an inability to collect biologic specimens and retention. Although this technology has interesting potential, it is unclear what type of research will be able to be performed using data collected using this platform.

## REGULATORY OVERSIGHT OF MEDICAL APPLICATIONS

With the proliferation of medical apps, it soon became clear that guidelines for regulatory oversight needed to be updated to keep pace with advances in technology. Currently, there is ambiguity in which apps constitute medical devices and how they should be regulated. In 2015, the Federal Trade Commission reached settlements with the makers of 2 apps, MelApp and Mole Detective, that purported to use images taken with a smartphone camera to determine if a mole was likely to be melanoma.[16] Because the Federal Trade Commission does not oversee medical devices, the basis of their claim was not on the medical safety of these apps but on the lack of evidence to support the claims made by these apps. To provide consistent regulatory oversight of apps for the safety of patients, the FDA published "Mobile Medical Applications: Guidance for Industry and Food and Drug Administration Staff,"[17] a document containing nonbinding recommendations, on February 9, 2015. This document states that regulatory oversight will be enforced on mobile apps that meet the definition of a medical device in the Federal Food, Drug and Cosmetic Act; are intended for use in performing a medical device function; and would cause harm to patients if it would not function properly. Fortunately, this document gives helpful guidance on the expected regulatory oversight that will be exercised for many of the types of apps discussed. Specifically, the document states that the FDA will exercise enforcement discretion regarding (ie, will not plan to regulate) "Apps specifically intended for medical uses that utilize the mobile device's built-in camera or a connected camera for purposes of documenting or transmitting pictures (eg, photos of a patient's skin lesions or wounds) to supplement or augment what would otherwise be a verbal description in a consultation between healthcare providers or between healthcare providers and patients/caregivers." This document also states, however, that "Mobile apps that analyze an image of a skin lesion using mathematical algorithms, such as fractal analysis, and provide the user with an assessment of the risk of the lesion" are an example of mobile apps that transform a smartphone into a regulated medical device and thus fall under the FDA's regulatory oversight.

Although this document provides some guidance, there are still open questions. For example, it is not clear what degree of oversight would apply to an app that uses a reference standard, such as a coin or color grid, to provide a patient with a measurement of the size and color of a lesion, particularly if it tracked changes in that lesion over time and thus provided some sort of even indirect assessment of risk. Additional questions are certain to arise as regulatory guidance struggles to keep pace with technologic advancement.

## ETHICAL ISSUES AND PRIVACY ISSUES OF SMARTPHONE APPLICATIONS

The increasingly widespread use of smartphone apps has posed new ethical challenges that need to be address if this new technology is to be fully realized with minimal risk of harm to patients. Although apps have the potential to enhance the delivery of health care, there are important ethical concerns regarding patient confidentiality, informed consent, transparency of data ownership, and data privacy protection. This is largely due to the fact that this rapidly evolving technology has outpaced the establishment of a system for regulatory oversight to certify a standard of care. Although guidelines have been delineated for the practice of high-quality teledermatology,[14] adherence to these standards is still purely voluntary.

According to one 2014 report, only 100 of 100,000 health care apps are FDA approved[18]; additionally, only approximately 12% of smartphone apps are HIPAA compliant.[19] Many apps require users to consent to their data policies, but how a patient's data are mined, used, and externally shared is often not transparent. The potential misuse of sensitive digital total body images is an area of vulnerability related to information safety and privacy and has become a growing area of concern, particularly when patient anonymity is not always possible.

Ownership of patients' health data collected through these apps is also unclear because developers of these technologies are not considered covered entities under HIPAA, and, as such, they are not legally obligated to protect a patient's health information. Thus, if a patient's digital photos are stored on a cloud server or disclosed to a third-party for the purposes of data analysis, liability becomes an issue if there is a privacy breach. Much like regulatory oversight, digital ethics surrounding medical apps are constantly evolving.

Also related to concerns over ownership and accountability are issues concerning medical licensure and malpractice liability, which present a significant challenge to the adoption of health care apps. For most teledermatology platforms, it is unclear how licensure regulations are enforced, particularly for teledermatologists practicing in a different state from the patients they are treating[20] or how malpractice liability would be determined if a patient were injured as a result of inaccurate information. This becomes even murkier if that inaccurate information is supplied not by a physician but by an automated algorithm that is part of a smartphone app.

Telemedicine has also fundamentally transformed the nature of the doctor-patient relationship. Despite its potential to bring about tremendous improvements and convenience, mobile health technology also carries with it a degree of depersonalization. As Gibbs[21] cautions, scientific advancements, although extremely important and valuable, are paradoxically providing diminishing returns for patients at the detriment of traditional doctor-patient relationships and healing arts.

## SUMMARY

Fifty years ago, Dr Albert Kligman, in a lecture entitled "Blind Man Dermatology," keenly asserted that "dermatology will enter the privileged domain of modern medicine when a blind man will not in the least be compromised in the practice or investigation of skin disease."[22] He challenged the field to develop a way for dermatologists to care for patients without reliance on the human eye. As smartphone apps become increasingly ubiquitous in health care, as Kourosh and Kvedar[23] describe, "dermatology has entered into a technological exploration phase, fashioning and testing innovations as predicted by a dermatologic Jules Verne decades ago."

The challenge for the field of dermatology is to balance the potential benefits of melanoma and skin cancer apps, including the ability to inexpensively provide education to the public and to provide access to dermatologists for patients who may otherwise go without expert care, with the potential harms they may pose, in particular the potential to provide false reassurance and thus delay the diagnosis of skin cancer. Potential app users should be made aware that currently there are no quality standards or regulatory oversight of medical apps. Ultimately, dermatologists' involvement in the development of apps for skin cancer diagnosis will help ensure that they are safe and effective and put the interest of patients first.

## REFERENCES

1. Anderson M. Technology device ownership: 2015. Pew research center. Available at: http://www.pewinternetorg/2015/10/29/technology-device-ownership-2015. Accessed May 12, 2016.
2. Hamilton AD, Brady RRW. Medical professional involvement in smartphone "apps" in dermatology. Br J Dermatol 2012;167(1):220–1.
3. March J, Hand M, Grossman D. Practical application of new technologies for melanoma diagnosis. J Am Acad Dermatol 2015;72(6):929–41.

4. Wolf JA, Moreau JF, Akilov O, et al. Diagnostic inaccuracy of smartphone applications for melanoma detection. JAMA Dermatol 2013;149(4):422–6.

5. Kassianos AP, Emery JD, Murchie P, et al. Smartphone applications for melanoma detection by community, patient and generalist clinician users: a review. Br J Dermatol 2015;172(6):1507–18.

6. Brewer AC, Endly DC, Henley J, et al. Mobile applications in dermatology. JAMA Dermatol 2013;149(11):1300.

7. Buller DB, Berwick M, Lantz K, et al. Smartphone mobile application delivering personalized, real-time sun protection advice. JAMA Dermatol 2015;151(5):497.

8. Buller DB, Berwick M, Lantz K, et al. Evaluation of immediate and 12-week effects of a smartphone sun-safety mobile application. JAMA Dermatol 2015;151(5):505.

9. Marek AJ, Chu EY, Ming ME, et al. Assessment of smartphone applications for total body digital photography-guided skin exams by patients. J Am Acad Dermatol 2016;75(5):1063–4.e1.

10. Uscher-Pines L, Malsberger R, Burgette L, et al. Effect of teledermatology on access to dermatology care among medicaid enrollees. JAMA Dermatol 2016. http://dx.doi.org/10.1001/jamadermatol.2016.0938.

11. Peart JM, Kovarik C. Direct-to-patient teledermatology practices. J Am Acad Dermatol 2015;72(5):907–9.

12. Finnane A, Dallest K, Janda M, et al. Teledermatology for the diagnosis and management of skin cancer. JAMA Dermatol 2016. http://dx.doi.org/10.1001/jamadermatol.2016.4361.

13. Resneck JS, Abrouk M, Steuer M, et al. Choice, Transparency, coordination, and quality among direct-to-consumer telemedicine websites and apps treating skin disease. JAMA Dermatol 2016;152(7):768.

14. Position Statement on Teledermatology. Available at: https://www.aad.org/Forms/Policies/Uploads/PS/PS-Teledermatology.pdf. Accessed March 1, 2017.

15. Wu X, Oliveria SA, Yagerman S, et al. Feasibility and efficacy of patient-initiated mobile teledermoscopy for short-term monitoring of clinically atypical nevi. JAMA Dermatol 2015;151(5):489–96.

16. FTC Cracks Down on Marketers of "Melanoma Detection" Apps, Federal Trade Commission. Available at: https://www.ftc.gov/news-events/press-releases/2015/02/ftc-cracks-down-marketers-melanoma-detection-apps. Accessed December 9, 2016.

17. Mobile Medical Applications: Guidance for Industry and Food and Drug Administration Staff. Available at: https://www.fda.gov/downloads/MedicalDevices/DeviceRegulationandGuidance/GuidanceDocuments/UCM263366.pdf. Accessed February 20, 2017.

18. Cortez NG, Cohen IG, Kesselheim AS, et al. FDA regulation of mobile health technologies. N Engl J Med 2014;371(4):372–9.

19. Anastasiou A, Giokas K, Koutsouris D. Monitoring of compliance on an individual treatment through mobile innovations. In: 37th Annual International Conference of the IEEE Engineering in Medicine and Biology Society (EMBC). Vol. 2015. IEEE. Milan (Italy): August 25–29, 2015. 7320–3.

20. Federation of State Medical Boards. Available at: https://www.fsmb.org/policy/advocacy-policy/key-issues. Accessed December 6, 2016.

21. Gibbs S. Losing touch with the healing art: dermatology and the decline of pastoral doctoring. J Am Acad Dermatol 2000;43(5):875–8.

22. Kligman A. Blind man dermatology. J Soc Cosmet Chem 1966;17:505–9.

23. Kourosh AS, Kvedar JC. Making mobile health measure up. JAMA Dermatol 2015;151(5):481–2.

# Teledermatology Applications in Skin Cancer Diagnosis

Frances M. Walocko, MSE, MD[a], Trilokraj Tejasvi, MBBS, MD[b],*

## KEYWORDS

- Teledermatology • Dermoscopy • Skin cancer • Pigmented lesions • Nonpigmented lesions
- Melanoma • Mobile teledermatology

## KEY POINTS

- Access to dermatologists for skin cancer screening is a growing problem.
- Teledermatology offers immediate skin cancer screening by transmitting medical information to a dermatologist for remote evaluation.
- Teledermatology has acceptable accuracy compared with a face-to-face clinical examination in diagnosing skin cancer and is a useful alternative for patients with poor access to health care.
- Addition of dermoscopy and/or reflectance confocal microscopy to a teledermatology consultation can help improve the diagnostic accuracy.

Skin cancer accounts for significant morbidity and mortality, and it is estimated that the value of life lost to society from melanoma ranges from $8 billion per year to $15 billion per year.[1,2] Early detection and treatment of these skin cancers could reduce the morbidity and mortality. The average wait time to see a dermatologist is 33.9 days.[3] This problem of access to a specialist could be partially resolved by using teledermatology. Teledermatology uses telecommunications to transmit medical information to a dermatologist for remote evaluation. Medical information may consist of clinical history, macroscopic photos, and/or dermoscopic images of skin lesions for remote evaluation. Teledermatology has drawn interest in the dermatologic community, because it allows for immediate and near comprehensive skin cancer screening for patients with poor access to health care.

The primary types of consultation using teledermatology include (1) synchronous, live interactive or (2) asynchronous, store-and-forward (**Table 1**). Live interactive consultation means that the patient and physician are able to interact with each other in real time. Store-and-forward consultation occurs when the patient's medical information is stored and then reviewed at a later time by a medical provider at a remote location (**Box 1**). Combining both live interactive and store-and-forward is called a hybrid consultation. The most common and successful type of consultation in teledermatology is store-and-forward. Consultations are generated either by a patient (direct to patient) or by another health care provider (consultative model). The latter is the most common and successful model, but consultations generated by patients are gaining popularity.

The authors do not have any commercial or financial conflicts of interest to disclose.

[a] University of Michigan Medical School, 1301 Catherine Street, Ann Arbor, MI 48109, USA; [b] Department of Dermatology, University of Michigan, 1910 Taubman Center, 1500 E. Medical Center Drive, Ann Arbor, MI 48109, USA

* Corresponding author.

E-mail address: ttejasvi@med.umich.edu

Dermatol Clin 35 (2017) 559–563
http://dx.doi.org/10.1016/j.det.2017.06.002
0733-8635/17/Published by Elsevier Inc.

**Table 1**
**Comparison of live interactive consultation versus store-and-forward consultation**

| Category | Live Interactive | Store-and-Forward |
|---|---|---|
| Description | Videoconferencing technology used for realtime interaction between patient and physician | Images and histories forwarded on to a consulting dermatologist |
| Physician-Patient Interaction | Allows for immediate advice and for the patient to ask questions | No interaction between patient and physician |
| Cost | Can be expensive due to videoconferencing technology | Relatively inexpensive |
| Convenience | Requires patient and physician to be available at same time | No need for coordinating scheduled visits; useful for patients with poor access to health care |
| Reimbursement | Yes | No |
| Internet speed | Highly dependent | Not dependent |
| Image quality | Lesser than still images | Superior images |

Digital photography is often used in a teledermatology consultation to replace visualization and touch.[4] The addition of dermoscopic images enhances the quality of the consultation. It also renders a high degree of confidence and accuracy in making a diagnosis, especially for a skin lesion.

**Box 1**
**Steps to perform a store-and-forward consultation**

Step 1: obtain a forest view, a close up view followed by a macroscopic image of the lesion[a]

↓

Step 2: wipe the lesion with an alcohol pad prior to taking dermoscopy images

↓

Step 3[b]: for cameras with only polarized dermoscope attachments (most commonly used): 2 modes

Noncontact mode – microscopic images taken less than 2 inches from the skin.

Contact mode – images taken while touching the skin.

For cameras with nonpolarized dermoscopy attachments: ultrasound gel or alcohol gel should be applied to reduce reflection from the skin surface; image should be taken while touching the skin.

[a]Please refer to ATA guidelines for instructions for taking these images: https://www.ncbi.nlm.nih.gov/pubmed/27690203.
[b]Newer photo-dermoscopy kits have both polarized and nonpolarized modes, which can be switched back and forth at the press of a button.

Dermoscopy, also known as dermatoscopy or epiluminescence microscopy, allows for noninvasive microscopic evaluation of skin lesions with a magnifying lens-like device. The images can then be digitized and transmitted electronically, which is known as teledermoscopy. This combination of digital photography and dermoscopy has the potential to improve skin cancer outcomes through early detection and management.

## HOW TO PERFORM A STORE-AND-FORWARD CONSULTATION FOR A SKIN LESION WITH DERMOSCOPY

Standard guidelines for performing a teledermatology store-and-forward consultation from the American Telemedicine Association are detailed by McKoy and colleagues[5] and can be obtained on the American Telemedicine Association Web site. Although there are no established standard practice guidelines for obtaining dermoscopy images, the authors recommend that a forest view followed by a close-up view and a macroscopic image of the lesion should be obtained in that order. The lesion is then to be wiped with an alcohol pad prior to taking dermoscopy images. For cameras with only polarized dermoscope attachments (most commonly used), microscopic images must be taken less than 2 inches from the skin (noncontact), followed by images taken while touching the skin (contact). For nonpolarized images, ultrasound gel or alcohol gel should be applied prior to contact with the lesion; this liquid interface reduces the reflection from the skin surface. Newer photo-dermoscopy kits have both polarized and nonpolarized modes that can be switched back and forth at the press of a button.

## TELEDERMATOLOGY FOR PIGMENTED LESIONS

Teledermatology has demonstrated acceptable concordance with standard face-to-face (FTF) clinical diagnosis in multiple settings for pigmented skin lesions concerning for melanoma. Piccolo and colleagues[6,7] compared diagnostic results of 66 pigmented skin lesions from macroscopic and dermatoscopic imaging with FTF clinical diagnosis. The authors found a concordance of 91% between teledermatology and FTF clinical diagnosis.[6,7] In another study conducted at the Minneapolis Veterans Affairs Medical Center Dermatology Clinic, 3021 skin lesions were reviewed, and an agreement between teledermatologists and clinical dermatologists was strong for aggregated diagnoses (primary diagnosis plus differential diagnoses) (78.6%-93.9%).[8] Arzberger and colleagues[9] compared teledermatology and FTF clinical diagnosis in a high-risk melanoma cohort using total-body photography, macroscopic images, and dermoscopic images of 1922 skin lesions. The general agreement, calculated by prevalence and bias-adjusted kappa (PABAK), showed almost perfect agreement (0.9–0.98).[9]

Diagnostic accuracy using teledermatology for pigmented skin lesions compared with the gold standard of histopathological diagnoses varies based on the type of skin lesion. Warshaw and colleagues[10] assessed accuracy of teledermatology and FTF clinical diagnoses compared with histopathological diagnoses and found greater accuracy for FTF clinical diagnoses compared with teledermatology for all categories of skin lesions. For dysplastic nevi, accuracy of teledermatology and FTF clinical diagnosis using macroscopic and polarized light dermoscopic images was 77.3% and 92.2%, respectively.[10] For melanoma, accuracy was 72.5% and 90.0%, respectively. For lentigines, diagnostic accuracy was 31.0% and 62.1%, respectively.[10] The group also noted that the accuracy of teledermatology and FTF clinical diagnoses seems to improve when more information is provided.[10] Use of dermoscopy in addition to macroscopic images led to greater accuracy compared with macroscopic images alone. Senel and colleagues[11] also directly assessed the impact of the addition of dermoscopy on the accuracy of teledermatologic diagnosis of nonmelanocytic lesions and found that dermoscopy significantly increased accuracy of diagnoses.

## TELEDERMATOLOGY FOR NONPIGMENTED LESIONS

Limited studies exist concerning reliability and accuracy of teledermatology for nonpigmented lesions compared with FTF clinical diagnoses and histopathological diagnoses. Senel and colleagues[11] evaluated a total of 150 patients with nonmelanocytic lesions and found a reliability of 0.86 and 0.88 (perfect agreement equals 1.0) for 2 teledermatologists compared with 2 clinical dermatologists. Accuracy of diagnoses when comparing the 2 teledermatologists to histopathological diagnoses was 88% and 95%, respectively.[11] Warshaw and colleagues[8] found that diagnostic agreement rates between teledermatologists and clinical dermatologists were higher for pigmented lesions (52.8%-93.9%) than nonpigmented lesions (47.7%-87.3%). Additional studies are needed to further evaluate the role of teledermatology in the diagnosis of nonpigmented lesions.

## LIMITATIONS OF TELEDERMATOLOGY

Despite the benefits of teledermatology for improving access to skin cancer screening and management, this technology has important limitations. One concern is the inability to complete full-body examinations on patients with concerning skin lesions. In a study completed by Viola and colleagues,[12] 149 cancerous lesions were noted in 98 patients.[12] However, only 88 cancers (59.1%) were identified in the index lesion; 111 incidental lesions were biopsied by the consulting dermatologist, and of those 111 lesions, 61 (55.0%) additional skin cancers were identified. The use of teledermatology to assess a specific lesion of concern may be associated with underdiagnosis of clinically significant lesions that are not appreciated by the referring physician. Another concerning factor is legal risks caused by diagnostic errors with teledermatology. To reduce complications from misdiagnosis, a conservative approach needs to be taken and specific training standards for dermoscopy need to be adopted. Lastly, some dermatologists have voiced concerns over the lack of patient-centric medicine that may result from telemedicine.

Many of these limitations and concerns may be outweighed by improved accessibility to dermatologists, earlier diagnosis of skin cancer, and patient satisfaction.[13,14] Teledermatology allows patients to address their individual medical concerns with a dermatologist in a timely manner, thereby creating a patient-centered approach to health care. Teledermatology networks have been implemented in areas of the world where patients have poor access to health care and have shown promising results. In 2004, a teledermatology network was implemented in Spain to connect 56 primary care centers with the skin cancer and melanoma clinic of a central hospital.[13] In the first 10 years,

43,677 patients were evaluated remotely. Breslow thickness in patients who had malignant melanoma managed through teledermatology was significantly thinner than that in patients whose referrals were conventionally managed.[13] In addition, a twofold increase in the detection rate of basal cell carcinoma was observed.[13] Another study in Spain involving 201 patients with primary cutaneous melanoma illustrated that the odds ratio of having a melanoma with a lower tumor stage was significantly higher in the teledermatology group compared with patients seen in clinic (odds ratio 1.96, 95% confidence interval [CI], 1.14–3.50; $P$ = .04).[15] In a separate study, Kahn and colleagues[16] demonstrated that the mean time to biopsy of skin cancer was 13.8 days for conventional referrals (median, 12.0 days) versus a mean of 9.7 days (median, 9.0 days) for teledermatology referrals ($P$<.0001) at California's Central Valley Kaiser Permanente. In addition, Livingstone and colleagues[14] point out that 97% of patients rated themselves as satisfied/very satisfied with their teledermatology experience; the median wait for the photos to be taken was 7 days, and 1 to 2 weeks for results.

## FUTURE DIRECTIONS: MOBILE TELEDERMATOLOGY AND REFLECTANCE CONFOCAL MICROSCOPY

Many technologies (covered elsewhere in this issue) are being applied to enhance teledermatology. As mobile technology continues to improve, smartphones have the potential to impact skin cancer screening and early detection. Mobile phones with built-in cameras and Internet connectivity can be used to transmit patient information from one provider to another through a secure application to facilitate remote diagnosis of skin conditions by dermatologists. In addition, dermatoscopes are available that can be mounted on the iPhone (Apple, Cupertino, California).[17] Cellular phone-based store-and-forward teledermatology has been applied as a triage tool in preliminary studies for skin cancer screening with acceptable diagnostic accuracy and agreement between the teledermatologist and an FTF clinical visit.[18–21]

In addition to using mobile phones to facilitate transmission of information between patients and physicians, various applications exist that use automated algorithms to analyze lesions found via self-skin examinations.[17] However, in a study comparing accuracy of applications for identifying concerning skin lesions, Wolf and colleagues[22] illustrated that applications with the highest sensitivity used a store-and-forward form of mobile teledermatology where the image was read by a remote dermatologist. Many smartphone-based applications may not be reliable for self-skin examinations when the image is not read by a trained teledermatologist.[17]

Overall, this technology is a supplement to regular total body skin examinations and does not serve as a replacement.[17] Mobile teledermatology restricts the clinical examination to individual lesions noticed by the patient, but the patient may have other concerning skin lesions only identifiable by a thorough skin examination. However, this technology is not designed to compare lesions to each other in order to identify the most atypical lesion on a patient.[17] Barriers also exist in terms of the degree of regulation by the US Food and Drug Administration (FDA) and guaranteeing that mobile applications are safe for patients to use.[17] Future advances in mobile teledermatology may address these concerns and increase the accuracy of self-skin examinations.

The other technology that is gaining popularity among some dermatologists is reflectance confocal microscopy (RCM). RCM is a noninvasive technique that helps ex vivo viewing and capturing high-resolution images of the cellular morphology. Studies have shown that the technique has high sensitivity to diagnose pigmented and nonpigmented lesions, but the specificity depends on training and expertise.[23,24] The cost and availability of the microscope are high and sparse, respectively. The expertise to analyze the images and educate the novice is gradually on the rise. More prospectively designed studies are required to make it safe and an affordable arm of teledermatology.[24]

## SUMMARY

In summary, teledermatology has made immediate screening of skin cancer possible in many places it would not be otherwise. Although teledermatology does not yet have the same diagnostic accuracy as traditional FTF clinical visits, it is a useful alternative for patients with poor access to specialty care. Creating more teledermatology networks in needed areas may significantly reduce the burden of dermatologic malignancies.

## ACKNOWLEDGMENTS

The authors thank Eric Arch for his help in preparation and submission of this article.

## REFERENCES

1. Federman DG, Kirsner RS, Viola KV. Skin cancer screening and primary prevention: facts and controversies. Clin Dermatol 2013;31(6):666–70.

2. Guy GP Jr, Machlin SR, Ekwueme DU, et al. Prevalence and costs of skin cancer treatment in the U.S., 2002-2006 and 2007-2011. Am J Prev Med 2015;48(2):183–7.

3. Coates SJ, Kvedar J, Granstein RD. Teledermatology: from historical perspective to emerging techniques of the modern era: part I: history, rationale, and current practice. J Am Acad Dermatol 2015; 72(4):563–74.

4. Bashshur RL, Shannon GW, Tejasvi T, et al. The empirical foundations of teledermatology: a review of the research evidence. Telemed J E Health 2015;21(12):953–79.

5. McKoy K, Antoniotti NM, Armstrong A, et al. Practice guidelines for teledermatology. Telemed J E Health 2016;22(12):981–90.

6. Piccolo D, Smolle J, Wolf IH, et al. Face-to-face diagnosis vs telediagnosis of pigmented skin tumors: a teledermoscopic study. Arch Dermatol 1999;135(12):1467–71.

7. Piccolo D, Smolle J, Argenziano G, et al. Teledermoscopy–results of a multicentre study on 43 pigmented skin lesions. J Telemed Telecare 2000;6(3): 132–7.

8. Warshaw EM, Gravely AA, Nelson DB. Reliability of store and forward teledermatology for skin neoplasms. J Am Acad Dermatol 2015;72(3):426–35.

9. Arzberger E, Curiel-Lewandrowski C, Blum A, et al. Teledermoscopy in high-risk melanoma patients: a comparative study of face-to-face and teledermatology visits. Acta Derm Venereol 2016;96(6):779–83.

10. Warshaw EM, Hillman YJ, Greer NL, et al. Teledermatology for diagnosis and management of skin conditions: a systematic review. J Am Acad Dermatol 2011;64(4):759–72.

11. Senel E, Baba M, Durdu M. The contribution of teledermatoscopy to the diagnosis and management of non-melanocytic skin tumours. J Telemed Telecare 2013;19(1):60–3.

12. Viola KV, Tolpinrud WL, Gross CP, et al. Outcomes of referral to dermatology for suspicious lesions: implications for teledermatology. Arch Dermatol 2011; 147(5):556–60.

13. Moreno-Ramirez D, Ferrandiz LA. 10-year history of teledermatology for skin cancer management. JAMA Dermatol 2015;151(12):1289–90.

14. Livingstone J, Solomon J. An assessment of the cost-effectiveness, safety of referral and patient satisfaction of a general practice teledermatology service. London J Prim Care (Abingdon) 2015;7(2): 31–5.

15. Ferrandiz L, Ruiz-de-Casas A, Martin-Gutierrez FJ, et al. Effect of teledermatology on the prognosis of patients with cutaneous melanoma. Arch Dermatol 2012;148(9):1025–8.

16. Kahn E, Sossong S, Goh A, et al. Evaluation of skin cancer in northern california kaiser permanente's store-and-forward teledermatology referral program. Telemed J E Health 2013;19(10):780–5.

17. March J, Hand M, Grossman D. Practical application of new technologies for melanoma diagnosis: part I. Noninvasive approaches. J Am Acad Dermatol 2015;72(6):929–41 [quiz: 941–2].

18. Massone C, Hofmann-Wellenhof R, Ahlgrimm-Siess V, et al. Melanoma screening with cellular phones. PLoS One 2007;2(5):e483.

19. Kroemer S, Frühauf J, Campbell T, et al. Mobile teledermatology for skin tumour screening: diagnostic accuracy of clinical and dermoscopic image tele-evaluation using cellular phones. Br J Dermatol 2011;164(5):973–9.

20. Lamel SA, Haldeman KM, Ely H, et al. Application of mobile teledermatology for skin cancer screening. J Am Acad Dermatol 2012;67(4):576–81.

21. Borve A, Terstappen K, Sandberg C, et al. Mobile teledermoscopy-there's an app for that! Dermatol Pract Concept 2013;3(2):41–8.

22. Wolf JA, Moreau JF, Akilov O, et al. Diagnostic inaccuracy of smartphone applications for melanoma detection. JAMA Dermatol 2013;149(4):422–6.

23. Farnetani F, Scope A, Braun RP, et al. Skin cancer diagnosis with reflectance confocal microscopy: reproducibility of feature recognition and accuracy of diagnosis. JAMA Dermatol 2015;151(10):1075–80.

24. Witkowski A, Łudzik J, Soyer HP. Telediagnosis with confocal microscopy: a reality or a dream? Dermatol Clin 2016;34(4):505–12.

# Integrating Skin Cancer–Related Technologies into Clinical Practice

Richard R. Winkelmann, DO[a], Aaron S. Farberg, MD[b],
Alex M. Glazer, MD[c], Clay J. Cockerell, MD[d], Arthur J. Sober, MD[e],
Daniel M. Siegel, MD, MS[f], Sancy A. Leachman, MD, PhD[g],
Whitney A. High, MD, JD[h], Orit Markowitz, MD[i], Brian Berman, MD, PhD[j],
David M. Pariser, MD[k], Gary Goldenberg, MD[l], Theodore Rosen, MD[m],
Darrell S. Rigel, MD, MS[n],*

## KEYWORDS

- Skin cancer • Technology • Diagnosis • Prognosis • Management • Melanoma • Dysplastic nevi
- Genetic testing

## KEY POINTS

- Early diagnosis and treatment of melanoma improve survival.
- New technologies are emerging that may augment the diagnosis, assessment, and management of melanoma but penetrance into everyday practice is low.
- In the current health care climate, greater emphasis will be placed on the incorporation of technology for clinically suspicious pigmented lesions to facilitate better, more cost-effective management.

Relevant Conflicts of Interest: Dr R.R. Winkelmann: fellowship funded in part by grant from Strata Skin Sciences Inc; Dr A.S. Farberg: fellowship funded in part by grant from Strata Skin Sciences Inc, consultant to Castle Biosciences Inc; Dr A.M. Glazer: participated in a research fellowship which was partially funded by Castle Biosciences Inc; Dr A.J. Sober: P.I for phase 4 Strata Skin Sciences Inc Trial; Dr C.J. Cockerell: consultant to Strata Skin Sciences Inc, Castle Biosciences Inc, and Myriad Genetics; Dr D.M. Siegel: member, Board of Directors, Caliber I.D.; Clinical Advisory Board, Michelson Diagnostics, LTD, and Advisory Board attendee for Castle Biosciences Inc; Dr S.A. Leachman: Myriad Genetics Laboratory Medical & Scientific Advisory Board member; Dr W. A. High: None; Dr O. Markowitz: consultant for 3-Gen, Michelson Diagnostics Ltd, and Strata Skin Sciences Inc; Dr B. Berman: None; Dr D.M. Pariser: Advisory Board attendee for Castle Biosciences Inc; Dr G. Goldenberg: consultant to Strata Skin Sciences Inc; Dr T. Rosen: Advisory Board attendee for Castle Biosciences Inc; and Dr D.S. Rigel: served as chief medical advisor to Strata Skin Sciences Inc, consultant to Castle Biosciences Inc.

[a] Department of Dermatology, OhioHealth, 75 Hospital Drive STE 250, Athens, OH 4570, USA; [b] Department of Dermatology, Icahn School of Medicine at Mt. Sinai, 1425 Madison Avenue, Floor 2, New York, NY 10029, USA; [c] National Society for Cutaneous Medicine, 35 East 35th Street #208, New York, NY 10016, USA; [d] Department of Dermatology, The University of Texas Southwestern Medical Center, 5939 Harry Hines Boulevard. 4th Floor, Suite 100, Dallas, TX 75390, USA; [e] Department of Dermatology, Harvard Medical School, 50 Staniford Street, 2nd Floor, Boston, MA 02114, USA; [f] Department of Dermatology, SUNY Downstate Medical Center, 450 Clarkson Avenue, Brooklyn, NY 11203, USA; [g] Department of Dermatology, OHSU Knight Cancer Institute, Oregon Health & Science University, 3303 S.W. Bond Avenue, Portland, OR 97239, USA; [h] Department of Dermatology & Pathology, University of Colorado School of Medicine, 12635 E Montview Boulevard, Bioscience Park, Suite 160, Aurora, CO 80045, USA; [i] Department of Dermatology, Mount Sinai Medical Center, 5 E 98th Street, FL 5, New York, NY 10029, USA; [j] Department of Dermatology, University of Miami Miller School of Medicine, 2925 Aventura Boulevard, Suite 205, Aventura, FL 33180, USA; [k] Department of Dermatology, Eastern Virginia Medical School, 6160 Kempsville Circle, Suite 200A, Norfolk, VA 23502, USA; [l] Department of Dermatology, Mount Sinai Medical Center, 5 E 98th Street, FL 5, New York, NY 10029, USA; [m] Department of Dermatology, Baylor College of Medicine, 1977 Butler Street, Suite E6.200, Houston, Texas 77030, USA; [n] Department of Dermatology, NYU School of Medicine, 35 East 35th Street #208, New York, NY 10016, USA
* Corresponding author.
E-mail address: dsrigel@prodigy.net

Dermatol Clin 35 (2017) 565–576
http://dx.doi.org/10.1016/j.det.2017.06.018

## INTRODUCTION

Currently, a vast majority of dermatologic diagnoses are made by visual inspection alone and/or dermoscopy, without the opportunity to enhance clinical examination with imaging or molecular tests. Several newer technologies, however, are available, Food and Drug Administration (FDA) approved, and proved efficacious aiding in the diagnosis and prognosis of melanoma.[1–44]

Despite the growing magnitude and dynamic evolution of research in this area, a recent survey reported only 11% of dermatologists even sometimes incorporate these emerging technologies into routine pigmented skin lesion (PSL) evaluation.[43] Given this low penetration, there seems to be a significant lack of knowledge related to these technologies and/or a material lack of understanding of how to appropriately integrate them into clinical practice. To help fill this knowledge gap and help clinicians better understand the rationale for and appropriate utilization of these new tools, the 11-member Melanoma Evolving Diagnostic Technologies Integration Group (MEDTIG) (Table 1) derived an algorithmic approach to systematically facilitate incorporating these technologies into the evaluation and management of suspicious PSLs. This algorithm is designed to serve as a template for clinicians to facilitate appropriate integration of these diagnostic and prognostic aids into their routine clinical practice.

## METHODS

A Medline search was performed for keywords (Melanoma, Diagnosis, Technology, Dysplastic Nevi, Genetic Testing, Prognosis, Imaging, and Molecular Testing) and 806 abstracts from January 1, 2012, to June 15, 2015, were considered. Additional earlier articles were selected when directly relevant to the scope of this article. After subsequent review, 49 articles of technologies with FDA approval and evidence-based efficacy were selected based on Oxford Centre for Evidence-Based Medicine criteria[44] and distributed to MEDTIG members. At a meeting on January 17, 2015, MEDTIG reviewed the best evidence pertaining to available methods for guiding decisions to biopsy suspicious PSLs, specimen evaluation, and melanoma risk stratification. Technologies that were not widely available, lacking support by strong translational studies, not FDA-approved, and/or in the process of validating their efficacy for melanoma diagnosis were not considered for inclusion in the algorithm. Technologies and their rationale for clinical utility have been described previously.[2,3] A summary of their mechanisms, efficacy, clinical utility, and estimated costs is

---

**Table 1**
**Eleven members of the Melanoma Evolving Diagnostic Technologies Integration Group**

| Panel Participant | Affiliation |
| --- | --- |
| Richard R. Winkelmann, DO | Cutaneous Oncology Clinical Research Fellow, National Society for Cutaneous Medicine, New York, NY |
| Clay J. Cockerell, MD | Clinical Professor of Dermatology, University of Texas Southwestern Medical Center, Dallas, TX |
| Arthur J. Sober, MD | Professor of Dermatology, Harvard Medical School, Boston, MA |
| Daniel M. Siegel, MD, MS | Clinical Professor of Dermatology, SUNY Downstate, Brooklyn, NY |
| Sancy A. Leachman, MD, PhD | Chair, Department of Dermatology, Oregon Health & Science University, Portland, OR |
| Whitney A. High, MD, JD | Associate Professor of Dermatology & Pathology, University of Colorado Denver School of Medicine, Aurora, CO |
| Orit Markowitz, MD | Assistant Professor of Dermatology, Mount Sinai Medical Center, New York, NY |
| Brian Berman, MD, PhD | Voluntary Professor of Dermatology, University of Miami Miller School of Medicine, Miami, FL |
| David M. Pariser, MD | Professor of Dermatology, Eastern Virginia Medical School, Norfolk, VA |
| Gary Goldenberg, MD | Assistant Clinical Professor of Dermatology, Mount Sinai Medical Center, New York, NY |
| Theodore Rosen, MD | Professor of Dermatology, Baylor College of Medicine, Houston, TX |
| Darrell S. Rigel, MD, MS | Department of Dermatology, New York University School of Medicine, New York, NY |

presented in **Table 2**. The algorithm was developed by consensus using a modified Delphi technique.[62] The Delphi technique has been effectively used in developing dermatologic expert panel recommendations to reach consensus.[45,63] Using this approach, a minimum of 70% agreement among participants was required to adopt a proposal. If 70% agreement could not be achieved, the proposal was returned to the group to be modified until the 70% agreement was achieved. After the adoption or rejection of each proposal, the algorithm was modified in real time and subject to discussion over the course of many rounds to reach consensus.

## RESULTS

The consensus-derived PSL evaluation and early management algorithm is presented in **Fig. 1**. The MEDTIG panel agreed that clinical, historical, and morphologic evaluation for asymmetry (A), border irregularity (B), color variegation (C), diameter greater than 6 mm (D),[64,65] and recent evolution (E),[66,67] patient concern (P), evidence of regression (R),[4] and "ugly duckling" signs (U)[68] (ABCDEPRU) is the first step in assessing a PSL of interest. Clinical evaluation should also include a thorough history to identify risk factors for melanoma, including personal/family history of melanoma, many atypical moles/ dysplastic nevi, genetic predisposition, childhood cancer history, immunosuppression, indoor tanning, blistering sunburns, Parkinson disease, and melanocortin-1 receptor genotype, if available.[4,69] Further examination with dermoscopy should be considered by clinicians with access to and adequate training in this diagnostic modality. Classification of the PSL based on clinical level of suspicion for diagnosis of melanoma or high-grade dysplastic nevus (HGDN) determines further evaluation and management. Through the use of the Delphi method, the MEDTIG panel reached consensus on the following criteria for melanoma suspicion: clinically high = greater than or equal to 90% suspicion, clinically intermediate = greater than 1% to less than 90% suspicion, and clinically low = less than or equal to 1% suspicion. Although the intermediate range may seem somewhat broad after initial clinical evaluation with the naked eye, an important aspect of the MEDTIG algorithm is the constant reassessment of PSL risk as additional information provided by the reviewed technologies is obtained. Additionally, the conservative nature of the initial risk assessment has been carefully determined to optimize patient care and minimize medicolegal risk based on the current state of evidence supporting the use of these technologies.

## Clinically High Suspicion Pigmented Skin Lesions

Tissue from these lesions should be sent for histologic evaluation. If the number of PSLs requiring biopsy exceeds what is reasonable and practical to perform in a single encounter, the MEDTIG panel–determined risk stratification should guide decisions on which PSLs to biopsy. Information provided by dermoscopy, reflectance confocal microscopy (RCM), and/or multispectral digital skin lesion analysis (MSDSLA) may be helpful for relative risk assessment and guide decisions on which PSLs to initially biopsy. The remaining lesions may be biopsied at a follow-up visit as appropriate.

All lesions identified as a melanoma or HGDN by histopathologic analysis require local excision. When histopathologic analysis for the diagnosis of melanoma or HGDN is equivocal, a dermatopathologist may supplement evaluation with 23-gene expression profiling (Dx23-GEP), immunohistochemistry (IHC), fluorescence in situ hybridization (FISH), and/or array-based comparative genomic hybridization (aCGH) testing. If these tests support or confirm a diagnosis of melanoma or HGDN, local excision is recommended.

After wide local excision of a primary melanoma, prognostic 31-gene expression profiling (Pr31-GEP) may be obtained to determine a patient's risk of distant metastasis. Patients identified as higher risk via Pr31-GEP testing may be considered for oncologic referral and sentinel lymph node biopsy (SLNBx), if not already performed. Lower-risk patients may be subject to observation/ follow-up appropriate for the diagnosis.

In line with the standard of care, after local excision of a melanoma, SLNBx can also be considered and discussed with patients having a Breslow thickness greater than or equal to 1.0 mm or less if additional negative prognostic factors exist (eg, ulceration and mitoses >1 mm²). If SLNBx is positive, oncologic referral is warranted for additional work-up and therapeutic or trial considerations. If SLNBx is negative, close observation/follow-up by a dermatologist or multispecialty group is recommended with consideration of oncologic referral for high-risk tumors or those greater than or equal to 1.0 mm in thickness. Pr31-GEP testing may also be considered regardless of SLNBx outcome because it may independently assess prognosis by revealing increased risk for metastatic disease.

**Table 2**
Summary of established and emerging technology information considered by the Melanoma Evolving Diagnostic Technologies Integration Group panel for algorithm recommendations

| Method/ Technology | Purpose | Description | Clinical Validation | Interpretation | Clinical Impact | Practical Considerations | Estimated Cost[b] | Level of Evidence[45] |
|---|---|---|---|---|---|---|---|---|
| Clinical examination | Identify suspicious PSLs with naked eye | Full-body skin examination | Sensitivity: 69% Specificity: 94%[11] | Subjective | First step in evaluating PSLs for risk and consideration for biopsy | • Efficient, cost-effective<br>• Limitations of naked eye and examiner expertise | | I |
| Dermoscopy | Evaluate suspicious PSLs | Uses 10× magnification with or without polarized light → pattern analysis | Sensitivity: 79%–93% Specificity: 69%–89%[46–52] | Subjective | Studies have shown increased sensitivity and specificity for detection of melanoma compared with naked-eye examination | • Ease of use, cost-efficient<br>• Requires specialized training to interpret accurately, may not enhance diagnosis of certain conditions | $300–$500 per device purchase | I |
| MSDSLA | Provides additional clinical information to enhance clinician biopsy decisions | Computerized imaging and analysis of 10 multispectral bandwidths (430–950 nm) up to 2.5 mm below the skin surface to measure degree of PSL morphologic disorganization | Sensitivity: 62%–98% Specificity: 10%–63%[17,18] | Objective | Aggregated data showed improvement in sensitivity, specificity, biopsy accuracy, negative predictive value, and positive predictive value with a decreased number of unnecessary biopsies | • Ease of use, analysis in < 3 s via handheld scanner, images to 2.5-mm depth<br>• Useful for evaluation of PSLs in cosmetically sensitive areas<br>• Individual cellular atypia is not visible at 20-μ resolution, higher costs | $100–$200 per sitting | II |

| | | | | | | |
|---|---|---|---|---|---|---|
| RCM | In vivo imaging allows for diagnosis and risk stratification | Uses a near-infrared 830-nm laser to image horizontal sections up to 300 μm in depth. Images can be captured sequentially to create 8 mm × 8 mm mosaic squares in a single horizontal plane at multiple levels of the epidermis and superficial dermis | Sensitivity: 91%–97% Specificity: 68%–86%[25,51-56] | Subjective | Has been shown to increase sensitivity, specificity, and biopsy accuracy compared with dermoscopy and clinical examination | • High resolution, in vivo imaging<br>• Useful for nonpigmented lesions<br>• Useful for evaluation of PSLs in cosmetically sensitive areas<br>• Requires specialized training to interpret, time-consuming, images to only 300 μm in depth, higher costs | $100 per lesion interpretation | — |
| Histo-pathology | Aids in diagnosis and staging | Method of staining and visualizing biopsied tissue under the microscope for interpretation by a dermatopathologist | No generalized systematic validation Favorable outcome accurately predicted in 47% of cases, unfavorable outcome accurately predicted in 73% of cases[55,57] | Subjective | Histopathologic assessment of melanoma is required for AJCC staging. It is extremely unlikely that a vast majority of institutions and insurers would proceed with care for melanoma in the absence of a histopathologic diagnosis, rendered and signed, by a licensed physician. | • Gold standard for melanoma diagnosis<br>• Can find significant discordance among examiners | $75–$150 per specimen | — |

(continued on next page)

**Table 2**
*(continued)*

| Method/ Technology | Purpose | Description | Clinical Validation | Interpretation | Clinical Impact | Practical Considerations | Estimated Cost[b] | Level of Evidence[45] |
|---|---|---|---|---|---|---|---|---|
| IHC[a] | Adjuvant to histopathology for diagnosis of MM in equivocal PSLs | Visualization of antigens on biopsied tissue specimen using catalyzed enzymes conjugated to antibodies | Sensitivity: 69%–100% Specificity: unknown[30,31,56] | Objective/ subjective | In PSLs with ambiguous or challenging histologic features IHC techniques may provide additional data to guide a final histologic interpretation | • Rapidity of investigations (IHC stains take only hours to perform) • Cost is relatively modest in comparison to other histopathologic adjunctive tests | $56–$100 per stain | II |
| aCGH | Adjuvant to histopathology for diagnosis of MM in equivocal PSLs | Method of analyzing copy number variations between entire genome of biopsied tissue and normal tissue controls | Sensitivity: 92%–96% Specificity: 87%–100%[57–60] | Objective | In lesions with ambiguous histologic features aCGH may provide additional data to guide management | • Requires a specimen with a relatively homogenous area of tumor cells of interest • Can only provide information on increased/ decreased copy numbers of genes • Longer turn-around time and generally higher costs than other adjunctive tests | $1200–$1800 per specimen | II |

| | | | | | | | |
|---|---|---|---|---|---|---|---|
| FISH | Allows identification of gene abnormalities on individual chromosomes typically using a 4-probe set with an internal control | Sensitivity: 43%–100% Specificity: 29%–80%[59–61] | Subjective | In lesions with ambiguous histologic features, FISH may provide additional data to guide management | • Can only provide information on increased/decreased copy numbers of genetic material for the probe set used<br>• Increased or decreased copy numbers outside of the probe set yields a false-negative result<br>• Tetraploidy yields a false-positive result | $600–$1000 per specimen | II |
| Dx23-GEP | Gene expression profiling using qRT-PCR to evaluate expression signature of 23 genes differentially expressed in malignant and benign PSLs | Sensitivity: 89%–90% Specificity: 91%–93%[39,40] | Objective | In lesions with ambiguous histologic features Dx23-GEP may provide additional data to guide management | • Validated on a relatively small set of PSLs that included only approxiamtley 10% spitzoid neoplasms<br>• Can be performed on unstained histopathology blocks<br>• Only used to differentiate between benign nevi and primary MM and subset of lesions cannot be differentiated | $150 cost to patient | II |

(continued on next page)

**Table 2**
*(continued)*

| Method/ Technology | Purpose | Description | Clinical Validation | Interpretation | Clinical Impact | Practical Considerations | Estimated Cost[b] | Level of Evidence[45] |
|---|---|---|---|---|---|---|---|---|
| Pr31-GEP | Assesses risk of metastasis in patients already diagnosed with MM | Gene expression profiling of isolated RNA via qRT-PCR measuring expression of 31 biomarkers within the tumor to classify stage I or II melanomas as low-risk (class 1) or high-risk (class 2) for future metastasis | Class 1 (lower metastatic risk subset): 79%–97% 5-y DFS Class 2 (higher metastatic risk subset): 31%–34% 5-y DFS[43,44] | Objective | Provides prognostic information for stages I and II melanomas. May identify persons at risk for metastatic disease independent of AJCC stage, Breslow depth, ulceration status, mitotic rate, and SLNBx status | • Potential to help triage patients being considered for SLNBx <br>• Requires tissue from the primary lesion <br>• Validated on a relatively small subset of PSLs <br>• Represents an additional step in management and additional cost | $200 cost to patient | II |

*Abbreviations:* AJCC, American Joint Committee on Cancer; BCC, basal cell carcinoma; DFS, disease-free survival; MM, malignant melanoma; qRT-PCR, quantitative reverse transcription–polymerase chain reaction.

[a] Sensitivity and specificity of IHC cannot be examined in the same manner as the other techniques in **Table 1**. Different IHC stains exist, and staining techniques vary among laboratories. Interpretation is both objective (present or absent) and subjective (a staining pattern). Most of the IHC sensitivity reported in the literature is simply the ability of the stain to mark melanocytes, whether benign or malignant. Specificity for distinguishing melanoma is largely unknown and/or debated. For example, some groups reported that affirmative expression of P16 makes a spitzoid neoplasm 8-fold more likely to be a Spitz nevus rather than melanoma, whereas other groups reported that P16 expression is of no utility in this distinction.

[b] Estimated costs in United States vary by region, health insurance plan, and overall financial status.

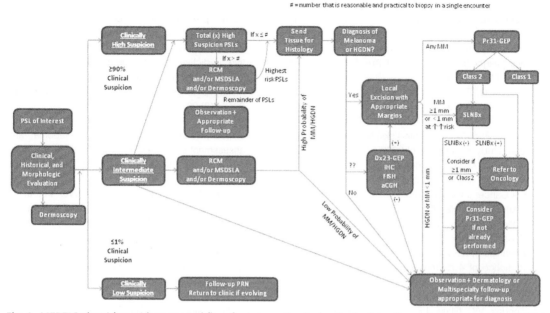

**Fig. 1.** MEDTIG algorithm with suggested flow for integrating technologies into diagnosis, assessment, and initial management of melanoma. MM, malignant melanoma; PRN, as needed.

## Clinically Intermediate Suspicion Pigmented Skin Lesions

PSLs of clinically intermediate suspicion may be further evaluated with dermoscopy and/or RCM and/or MSDSLA if available. If any of these diagnostic modalities determines a clinically intermediate suspicion PSL has a high probability of being melanoma or an HGDN, biopsy is recommended as long as the total number of biopsies remains less than what is reasonable and practical for a single office encounter. For clinically intermediate suspicion PSLs in which the probability of being a melanoma or HGDN is subsequently determined to be low, observation/follow-up appropriate for the diagnosis is recommended. If newer technologies are not available to aid the evaluation of clinically intermediate suspicion PSLs, the clinician may decide to send the lesion for histologic evaluation or elect for observation/follow-up as appropriate.

## Clinically Low Suspicion Pigmented Skin Lesions

PSLs identified clinically to be of low suspicion should not require intervention. Patients should be advised, however, to follow-up on an as-needed basis, returning for evaluation if the PSL is evolving.

## SUMMARY

The continued rising incidence of melanoma creates an increasing need for strategies that can improve early detection and enhance subsequent appropriate management. Since the advent of the asymmetry, boarder, color, diameter (ABCDs) of early melanoma 30 years ago, technologies have been developed to augment the evaluation of PSLs. Advanced molecular genetic tests have also evolved as adjuncts to standard pathology techniques for improving melanoma diagnosis and for risk stratification of melanoma patients. Currently, the availability of these technologies is still somewhat limited and their potential overall impact on melanoma has not yet been achieved. Access to these technologies, however, will grow and there is already sufficient evidence to justify their implementation in clinical practice. The MED-TIG workflow algorithm presented in this article is intended to fill a demonstrated knowledge gap by providing dermatologists with a systematic approach to effectively integrate these diagnostic and prognostic technologies into melanoma diagnosis and early management, thereby potentially improving clinical efficiency and overall patient outcomes. MEDTIG expects this algorithm should be revisited in several years as more studies yield additional data and new technologies emerge.

## REFERENCES

1. March J, Hand M, Grossman D. Practical application of new technologies for melanoma diagnosis: Part I. Noninvasive approaches. J Am Acad Dermatol 2015;72(6):929–41.

2. Mayer JE, Swetter SM, Fu T, et al. Screening, early detection, education, and trends for melanoma: Current status (2007-2013) and future directions. Part I. Epidemiology, high-risk groups, clinical strategies, and diagnostic technology. J Am Acad Dermatol 2014;71:599.e1-12.

3. Piccolo D, Ferrari A, Peris K, et al. Dermoscopic diagnosis by a trained clinician vs. a clinician with minimal dermoscopy training vs. computer-aided diagnosis of 341 pigmented skin lesions: a comparative study. Br J Dermatol 2002;147(3):481–6.

4. Rigel DS, Russak J, Friedman R. The evolution of melanoma diagnosis: 25 years beyond the ABCDs. CA Cancer J Clin 2010;60:301–16.

5. Markowitz O. Handbook on dermoscopy: a color wheel approach. 1st edition. Philadelphia: Lippincott Williams & Wilkins; 2016.

6. Dolianitis C, Kelly J, Wolfe R, et al. Comparative performance of 4 dermoscopic algorithms by nonexperts for the diagnosis of melanocytic lesions. Arch Dermatol 2005;141(8):1008–14.

7. Sondak VK, Glass LF, Geller AC. Risk-stratified screening for detection of melanoma. JAMA 2015; 313(6):616–7.

8. Kellner C, Reinhold U. Modern diagnostic procedures in dermatological oncology. Pathologe 2015; 36(1):11–5.

9. Shoo BA, Sagebiel RW, Kashani-Sabet M. Discordance in the histopathologic diagnosis of melanoma at a melanoma referral center. J Am Acad Dermatol 2010;62(5):751–6.

10. Vestergaard ME, Macaskill P, Holt PE, et al. Dermoscopy compared with naked eye examination for the diagnosis of primary melanoma: a meta-analysis of studies performed in a clinical setting. Br J Dermatol 2008;159(3):669–76.

11. Thomas NE, Kricker A, Waxweiler WT, et al. Comparison of clinicopathologic features and survival of histopathologically amelanotic and pigmented melanomas. JAMA Dermatol 2014;150(12):1306–14.

12. Skvara H, Teban L, Fiebiger M, et al. Limitations of dermoscopy in the recognition of melanoma. Arch Dermatol 2005;141(2):155–60.

13. Mascolo M, Russo D, Scalvenzi M, et al. Pitfalls in the dermoscopic diagnosis of amelanotic melanoma. J Am Acad Dermatol 2015;72(1 Suppl): S2–3.

14. Elbaum M, Kopf AW, Rabinovitz HS, et al. Automatic differentiation of melanoma and melanocytic nevi with multispectral digital dermoscopy: a feasibility study. J Am Acad Dermatol 2001;44(2): 207–18.

15. Monheit G, Cognetta AB, Ferris L, et al. The performance of MelaFind: a prospective multicenter study. Arch Dermatol 2011;147(2):188–94.

16. Winkelmann RR, Tucker N, White R, et al. Evaluating diagnostic enhancement with multi-spectral digital skin lesion analysis: a meta-analysis of 5 studies. Poster presentation: Winter Clinical Dermatology Conference. Kaanapali (HI), January 16–21, 2014.

17. Winkelmann RR, Rigel DS, Kollmann E, et al. Negative predictive value of pigmented lesion evaluation by multispectral digital skin lesion analysis in a community practice setting. J Clin Aesthet Dermatol 2015;8(3):20–2.

18. Busam KJ, Hester K, Charles C, et al. Detection of clinically amelanotic malignant melanoma and assessment of its margins by in vivo confocal scanning laser microscopy (CSLM). Arch Dermatol 2001; 137(7):923–9.

19. Langley RG, Rajadhyaksha M, Dwyer PJ, et al. Confocal scanning laser microscopy of benign and malignant melanocytic skin lesions in vivo. J Am Acad Dermatol 2001;45(3):365–76.

20. Charles CA, Marghoob AA, Busam KJ, et al. Melanoma or pigmented basal cell carcinoma: a clinical-pathologic correlation with dermoscopy, in vivo confocal scanning laser microscopy, and routine histology. Skin Res Technol 2002;8(4):282–7.

21. Stevenson AR, Mickan S, Mallett S, et al. Systematic review of diagnostic accuracy of reflectance confocal microscopy for melanoma diagnosis in patients with clinically equivocal skin lesions. Dermatol Pract Concept 2013;3(4):19–27.

22. Pellacani G, Pepe P, Casari A, et al. Reflectance confocal microscopy as a second-level examination in skin oncology improves diagnostic accuracy and saves unnecessary excisions: a longitudinal prospective study. Br J Dermatol 2014; 171(5):1044–51.

23. Guitera P, Pellacani G, Longo C, et al. In vivo reflectance confocal microscopy enhances secondary evaluation of melanocytic lesions. J Invest Dermatol 2009;129(1):131–8.

24. Van Dijk MC, Aben KK, van Hees F. Expert review remains important in the histological diagnosis of cutaneous melanocytic lesions. Histopathology 2008; 52(2):139–46.

25. Veenhuizen KC, De Wit PE, Mooi WJ, et al. Quality assessment by expert opinion in melanoma pathology: experience of the pathology panel of the Dutch Melanoma Working Party. J Pathol 1997;182(3): 266–72.

26. Farmer ER, Gonin R, Hanna MP. Discordance in the histopathologic diagnosis of melanoma and melanocytic nevi between expert pathologists. Hum Pathol 1996;27(6):528–31.

27. Suarez A, High WA. Principles of molecular diagnostics and personalized cancer medicine. In: Chapter 34: immunohistochemical and molecular diagnosis of melanoma. 1st edition. Philadelphia: Lippincott Williams & Winkins; 2013. p. 434–50.

28. George E, Polissar NL, Wick M. Immunohistochemical evaluation of p16INK4A, E-cadherin, and cyclin

D1 expression in melanoma and Spitz tumors. Am J Clin Pathol 2010;133:370–9.

29. Mason A, Wititsuwannakul J, Klump VR, et al. Expression of p16 alone does not differentiate between Spitz nevi and Spitzoid melanoma. J Cutan Pathol 2012;39:1062–74.

30. Gerami P, Busam KJ. Cytogenetic and mutational analyses of melanocytic tumors. Dermatol Clin 2012;30(4):555–66.

31. Neogenomics, Inc NeoSITE™ Melanoma: next-Generation FISH analysis for ambiguous melanocytic lesions. Available at: http://www.neogenomics.com/neosite-melanoma.htm. Accessed June 18, 2015.

32. Tetzlaff MT, Wang WL, Milless TL, et al. Ambiguous melanocytic tumors in a tertiary referral center: the contribution of fluorescence in situ hybridization (FISH) to conventional histopathologic and immunophenotypic analyses. Am J Surg Pathol 2013;37:1783–96.

33. Kerl K, Palmedo G, Wiesner T, et al. A proposal for improving multicolor FISH sensitivity in the diagnosis of malignant melanoma using new combined criteria. Am J Dermatopathol 2012;34:580–5.

34. Zembowicz A, Yang SE, Kafanas A, et al. Correlation between histologic assessment and fluorescence in situ hybridization using MelanoSITE in evaluation of histologically ambiguous melanocytic lesions. Arch Pathol Lab Med 2012;136(12):1671–9.

35. North JP, Vemula SS, Bastian BC. Chromosomal copy number analysis in melanoma diagnostics. Methods Mol Biol 2014;1102:199–226.

36. Ali L, Helm T, Cheney R, et al. Correlating array comparative genomic hybridization findings with histology and outcome in spitzoid melanocytic neoplasms. Int J Clin Exp Pathol 2010;3:593–9.

37. Clark LE, Warf MB, Flake DD, et al. Clinical validation of a gene expression signature that differentiates benign nevi from malignant melanoma. J Cutan Pathol 2015;42(4):244–52.

38. Clarke LE, Berking C, Tahan S, et al. Development of a gene expression signature to differentiate malignant melanoma from benign melanocytic nevi. Poster presentation: Society for Melanoma Research International Congress. Philadelphia, November 17–19, 2013.

39. Clarke LE, Bess E, Kolquist K, et al. A clinically validated gene expression score impacts diagnosis and management recommendations of melanocytic lesions by dermatopathologists. Poster presentation: College of American Pathologists Meeting. Chicago, September 7–10, 2014.

40. Lawson DH, Russell M, Wilkinson J, et al. Gene expression profile of primary cutaneous melanomas to distinguish between low and high risk of metastasis. J Clin Oncol 2013;31:s9022.

41. Gerami P, Cook RW, Wilkinson J, et al. Development of a prognostic genetic signature to predict the metastatic risk associated with melanoma. Clin Cancer Res 2015;21(1):175–81.

42. Gerami P, Cook RW, Russell MC, et al. Gene expression profiling for molecular staging of cutaneous melanoma in patients with sentinel lymph node biopsy. J Am Acad Dermatol 2015;72(5):780–5.e3.

43. Winkelmann RR, Rigel DS. Summary of dermatologist assessment and management of dysplastic nevi: a follow-up survey. J Am Acad Dermatol 2015;73(6):27–9.

44. Oxford Center for Evidence Based Medicine. Available at: http://www.cebm.net/index.aspx?o=5653. Accessed December 20, 2016.

45. Richard MA, Barnetche T, Rouzaud M, et al. Evidence-based recommendations on the role of dermatologists in the diagnosis and management of psoriatic arthritis: systematic review and expert opinion. J Eur Acad Dermatol Venereol 2014;28s5:3–12.

46. Argenziano G, Puig S, Zalaudek I, et al. Dermoscopy improves accuracy of primary care physicians to triage lesions suggestive of skin cancer. J Clin Oncol 2006;24:1877–82.

47. Bono A, Bartoli C, Cascinelli N, et al. Melanoma detection. A prospective study comparing diagnosis with the naked eye, dermatoscopy and telespectrophotometry. Dermatology 2002;205:362–6.

48. Bono A, Tolomio E, Trincone S, et al. Micro-melanoma detection: a clinical study on 206 consecutive cases of pigmented skin lesions with a diameter < or = 3 mm. Br J Dermatol 2006;155:570–3.

49. Cristofolini M, Zumiani G, Bauer P, et al. Dermatoscopy: usefulness in the differential diagnosis of cutaneous pigmentary lesions. Melanoma Res 1994;4:391–4.

50. Benelli C, Roscetti E, Dal Pozzo V, et al. The dermoscopic versus the clinical diagnosis of melanoma. Eur J Dermatol 1999;9:470–6.

51. Curchin CES, Wurm EMT, Lambie DLJ, et al. First experiences using reflectance confocal microscopy on equivocal skin lesions in Queensland. Australas J Dermatol 2011;52:89–97.

52. Guitera P, Pellacani G, Crotty KA, et al. The impact of in vivo reflectance confocal microscopy on the diagnostic accuracy of lentigo maligna and equivocal pigmented and nonpigmented macules of the face. J Invest Dermatol 2010;130:2080–91.

53. Pellacani G, Guitera P, Longo C, et al. The impact of in vivo reflectance confocal microscopy for the diagnostic accuracy of melanoma and equivocal melanocytic lesions. J Invest Dermatol 2007;127:2759–65.

54. Langley RG, Walsh N, Sutherland AE, et al. The diagnostic accuracy of in vivo confocal scanning laser microscopy compared to dermoscopy of benign and malignant melanocytic lesions: A prospective study. Dermatology 2007;215:365–72.

55. Cerroni L, Barnhill R, Elder D, et al. Melanocytic tumors of uncertain malignant potential: results of a tutorial held at the XXIX Symposium of the International Society of Dermatopathology in Graz, October 2008. Am J Surg Pathol 2010;34: 314–26.

56. Ohsie SJ, Sarantopoulos GP, Cochran AJ, et al. Immunohistochemical characteristics of melanoma. J Cutan Pathol 2008;35:433–44.

57. Bastian BC, Olshen AB, LeBoit PE, et al. Classifying melanocytic tumors based on DNA copy number changes. Am J Pathol 2003;163:1765–70.

58. Wang L, Rao M, Fang Y, et al. A genome-wide high resolution array CGH analysis of cutaneous melanoma and comparison of aCGH to FISH in diagnostic evaluation. J Mol Diagn 2013;15: 581–91.

59. Gerami P, Jewell SS, Morrison LE, et al. Fluorescence in situ hybridization (FISH) as an ancillary diagnostic tool in the diagnosis of melanoma. Am J Surg Pathol 2009;33:1146–56.

60. Gaiser T, Kutzner H, Palmedo G, et al. Classifying ambiguous melanocytic lesions with FISH and correlation with clinical long-term follow up. Mod Pathol 2010;23:413–9.

61. Vergier B, Prochazkova-Carlotti M, de la Fouchardiere A, et al. Fluorescence in situ hybridization, a diagnostic aid in ambiguous melanocytic tumors: European study of 113 cases. Mod Pathol 2011;24:613.

62. Sanford BA, Chia-Chien H. The Delphi technique: making sense of consensus. Practical Assessment, Research & Evaluation 2007;12(10):1–8.

63. Gottlieb AB, Levin AA, Armstrong AW, et al. The International Dermatology Outcome Measures Group: formation of patient-centered outcome measures in dermatology. J Am Acad Dermatol 2015;72(2):345–8.

64. Friedman RJ, Rigel DS, Kopf AW. Early detection of malignant melanoma: the role of physician examination and self-examination of the skin. CA Cancer J Clin 1985;35(3):130–51.

65. Rigel DS, Friedman RJ. The rationale of the ABCDs of early melanoma. J Am Acad Dermatol 1993;29: 1060–1.

66. Kopf AW, Welkovich B, Frankel RE, et al. Thickness of malignant melanoma: global analysis of related factors. J Dermatol Surg Oncol 1987;13:345–90, 401–20.

67. Abbasi NR, Shaw HM, Rigel DS, et al. Early diagnosis of cutaneous melanoma: revisiting the ABCD criteria. JAMA 2004;292:2771–6.

68. Scope A, Dusza SW, Halpern AC, et al. The "ugly duckling" sign: agreement between observers. Arch Dermatol 2008;144(1):58–64.

69. March J, Hand M, Truong A, et al. Practical application of new technologies for melanoma diagnosis: Part II. Molecular approaches. J Am Acad Dermatol 2015;72(6):943–58.

# UNITED STATES POSTAL SERVICE ®
## Statement of Ownership, Management, and Circulation (All Periodicals Publications Except Requester Publications)

| 1. Publication Title | 2. Publication Number | 3. Filing Date |
|---|---|---|
| DERMATOLOGIC CLINICS | 000 – 705 | 9/18/2017 |

| 4. Issue Frequency | 5. Number of Issues Published Annually | 6. Annual Subscription Price |
|---|---|---|
| JAN, APR, JUL, OCT | 4 | $377.00 |

7. Complete Mailing Address of Known Office of Publication (Not printer) (Street, city, county, state, and ZIP+4®)

ELSEVIER INC.
230 Park Avenue, Suite 800
New York, NY 10169

Contact Person
STEPHEN R. BUSHING

Telephone (Include area code)
215-239-3688

8. Complete Mailing Address of Headquarters or General Business Office of Publisher (Not printer)

ELSEVIER INC.
230 Park Avenue, Suite 800
New York, NY 10169

9. Full Names and Complete Mailing Addresses of Publisher, Editor, and Managing Editor (Do not leave blank)

Publisher (Name and complete mailing address)

ADRIANNE BRIGIDO, ELSEVIER INC.
1600 JOHN F KENNEDY BLVD. SUITE 1800
PHILADELPHIA, PA 19103-2899

Editor (Name and complete mailing address)

JESSICA MCCOOL, ELSEVIER INC.
1600 JOHN F KENNEDY BLVD. SUITE 1800
PHILADELPHIA, PA 19103-2899

Managing Editor (Name and complete mailing address)

PATRICK MANLEY, ELSEVIER INC.
1600 JOHN F KENNEDY BLVD. SUITE 1800
PHILADELPHIA, PA 19103-2899

10. Owner (Do not leave blank. If the publication is owned by a corporation, give the name and address of the corporation immediately followed by the names and addresses of all stockholders owning or holding 1 percent or more of the total amount of stock. If not owned by a corporation, give the names and addresses of the individual owners. If owned by a partnership or other unincorporated firm, give its name and address as well as those of each individual owner. If the publication is published by a nonprofit organization, give its name and address.)

| Full Name | Complete Mailing Address |
|---|---|
| WHOLLY OWNED SUBSIDIARY OF REED/ELSEVIER US HOLDINGS | 1600 JOHN F KENNEDY BLVD. SUITE 1800 PHILADELPHIA, PA 19103-2899 |

11. Known Bondholders, Mortgagees, and Other Security Holders Owning or Holding 1 Percent or More of Total Amount of Bonds, Mortgages, or Other Securities. If none, check box ➤ ☐ None

| Full Name | Complete Mailing Address |
|---|---|
| N/A | |

12. Tax Status (For completion by nonprofit organizations authorized to mail at nonprofit rates) (Check one)
The purpose, function, and nonprofit status of this organization and the exempt status for federal income tax purposes:
☒ Has Not Changed During Preceding 12 Months
☐ Has Changed During Preceding 12 Months (Publisher must submit explanation of change with this statement)

| 13. Publication Title | 14. Issue Date for Circulation Data Below |
|---|---|
| DERMATOLOGIC CLINICS | JULY 2017 |

| 15. Extent and Nature of Circulation | | Average No. Copies Each Issue During Preceding 12 Months | No. Copies of Single Issue Published Nearest to Filing Date |
|---|---|---|---|
| a. Total Number of Copies (Net press run) | | 365 | 232 |
| b. Paid Circulation (By Mail and Outside the Mail) | (1) Mailed Outside-County Paid Subscriptions Stated on PS Form 3541 (Include paid distribution above nominal rate, advertiser's proof copies, and exchange copies) | 98 | 91 |
| | (2) Mailed In-County Paid Subscriptions Stated on PS Form 3541 (Include paid distribution above nominal rate, advertiser's proof copies, and exchange copies) | 0 | 0 |
| | (3) Paid Distribution Outside the Mails Including Sales Through Dealers and Carriers, Street Vendors, Counter Sales, and Other Paid Distribution Outside USPS® | 72 | 74 |
| | (4) Paid Distribution by Other Classes of Mail Through the USPS (e.g. First-Class Mail®) | 0 | 0 |
| c. Total Paid Distribution [Sum of 15b (1), (2), (3), and (4)] | | 170 | 165 |
| d. Free or Nominal Rate Distribution (By Mail and Outside the Mail) | (1) Free or Nominal Rate Outside-County Copies included on PS Form 3541 | 70 | 67 |
| | (2) Free or Nominal Rate In-County Copies Included on PS Form 3541 | 0 | 0 |
| | (3) Free or Nominal Rate Copies Mailed at Other Classes Through the USPS (e.g. First-Class Mail) | 0 | 0 |
| | (4) Free or Nominal Rate Distribution Outside the Mail (Carriers or other means) | 0 | 0 |
| e. Total Free or Nominal Rate Distribution (Sum of 15d (1), (2), (3) and (4)) | | 70 | 67 |
| f. Total Distribution (Sum of 15c and 15e) | | 240 | 232 |
| g. Copies not Distributed (See Instructions to Publishers #4 (page #3)) | | 125 | 0 |
| h. Total (Sum of 15f and g) | | 365 | 232 |
| i. Percent Paid (15c divided by 15f times 100) | | 70.83% | 71.12% |

* If you are claiming electronic copies, go to line 16 on page 3. If you are not claiming electronic copies, skip to line 17 on page 3.

| 16. Electronic Copy Circulation | Average No. Copies Each Issue During Preceding 12 Months | No. Copies of Single Issue Published Nearest to Filing Date |
|---|---|---|
| a. Paid Electronic Copies | 0 | 0 |
| b. Total Paid Print Copies (Line 15c) + Paid Electronic Copies (Line 16a) | 170 | 165 |
| c. Total Print Distribution (Line 15f) + Paid Electronic Copies (Line 16a) | 240 | 232 |
| d. Percent Paid (Both Print & Electronic Copies) (16b divided by 16c × 100) | 70.83% | 71.12% |

☒ I certify that 50% of all my distributed copies (electronic and print) are paid above a nominal price.

17. Publication of Statement of Ownership
☒ If the publication is a general publication, publication of this statement is required. Will be printed in the _____ OCTOBER 2017 _____ issue of this publication. ☐ Publication not required.

18. Signature and Title of Editor, Publisher, Business Manager, or Owner

*Stephen R. Bushing*   Date 9/18/2017

STEPHEN R. BUSHING - INVENTORY DISTRIBUTION CONTROL MANAGER

I certify that all information furnished on this form is true and complete. I understand that anyone who furnishes false or misleading information on this form or who omits material or information requested on the form may be subject to criminal sanctions (including fines and imprisonment) and/or civil sanctions (including civil penalties).

PS Form **3526**, July 2014 (Page 3 of 4)   PRIVACY NOTICE: See our privacy policy on www.usps.com.

PS Form **3526**, July 2014 (Page 1 of 4 (see instructions page 4))   PSN 7530-01-000-9631   PRIVACY NOTICE: See our privacy policy on www.usps.com.

# Moving?

## Make sure your subscription moves with you!

To notify us of your new address, find your **Clinics Account Number** (located on your mailing label above your name), and contact customer service at:

**Email: journalscustomerservice-usa@elsevier.com**

**800-654-2452** (subscribers in the U.S. & Canada)
**314-447-8871** (subscribers outside of the U.S. & Canada)

**Fax number: 314-447-8029**

**Elsevier Health Sciences Division**
**Subscription Customer Service**
**3251 Riverport Lane**
**Maryland Heights, MO 63043**

ELSEVIER

Printed and bound by CPI Group (UK) Ltd, Croydon, CR0 4YY

03/10/2024

01040383-0014